Big to Small

Clean Eating for Successful Weight Loss

Martin Foster

a licensed professional before attempting any techniques outlined in this book.

By reading this document, the reader agrees that under no circumstances is the author responsible for any losses, direct or indirect, that are incurred as a result of the use of the information contained within this document, including, but not limited to, errors, omissions, or inaccuracies.

Table of Contents

Introduction

The various restraints and uncertainties can be overwhelming when looking for the perfect diet and exercise regime. For example, what is the best food to lose weight the fastest? How much am I allowed to eat on a given day? When do I eat what? Do I at least get a cheat day? How long do I have to do this? You will surely ask yourself these questions when searching for the perfect plan. These questions are also answered in *Big to Small: Clean Eating for Successful Weight Loss*. In addition, the program will go over each step to ensure success in achieving your weight loss goals, or, as I like to say, your "health gain goals."

The point that hooked me to the idea of the ketogenic diet was the fact that food can heal our insecurities. Instead of buying endless amounts of weight loss pills and trying out multiple fad diets, I was hooked onto the idea of a ketogenic diet and its everlasting effects without changing my lifestyle forever.

To accomplish anything, you need to be prepared. I will show you some of my quick tips to keep to the ketogenic, or keto, diet and explain why I wrote this book. I was tired of taking various pills and destroying my gut with these pharmaceutical replacements, so I decided to look elsewhere. After my first keto cycle, I felt like a baby bird breaking out of my shell for the first time. There were lots of days when I felt more like I was knee deep in quicksand, but they passed quickly, and the results were inexplicable.

From personal experience, I can ensure your success in this program. I struggled trying to find a healthy, delicious, and doable diet. I am fit and exercise regularly, but I struggled over the years to maintain a consistent weight alongside a healthy diet that fueled my needs more than it fueled my desire to lose weight. The basic overview involves a keto-based diet, a few days of exercise each week, and some personal tricks and tools to use through the next three weeks. A great idea is to keep a daily journal of how you feel, what you've eaten, and the changes occurring in your body, moods, emotions, and progress, and then going back and reading them when you're having a hard day. Progress is what promotes success, whereas defeat is easier and more alluring than fighting back. So, when you've had bad days, it's good to get those feelings out and be heard in some way. But, when you're feeling strong, powerful, and ready, you can look back on those thoughts and that mindset to get you through the former.

The *Big to Small* keto diet plan outlined in this book has been perfected over time and contains simple, yet effective rules for you to follow. Using these keto-friendly ingredients and flavorful recipes will assure that you eat what you need to lose weight and feel great. In addition, the brief, convenient exercise suggestions are doable wherever and whenever you can squeeze them into your busy schedule.

Before you jump in, know that you'll experience some detoxifying symptoms. This occurs because you're eliminating and depriving your body of one of its major sources of energy. Once you work through those couple of days, it will be a breeze. I would suggest starting on a Wednesday to avoid experiencing any negative symptoms at work in the middle of the workweek. You could also start your day with a cup of warm water with lemon and a teaspoon of baking soda which will help with these symptoms. This basically due to the fact most meats contain purines that turn to uric acid in the body. High levels of uric acid could cause symptoms like fatigue, trouble sleeping, muscle weakness, and body aches (Berg, 2017). But, when you drink citric acid like that found in lemons, your body turns that into an alkaline which then helps neutralize that uric acid. Therefore, I suggest adding lemons to your keto diet, especially if you're doing it frequently, because an excess of uric acid can lead to serious issues. In fact, adding lemon to any diet is beneficial because of the quantity of foods in everyday diets that cause high buildups of uric acid, such as beer, game meats, sardines, herring, and coffee.

Why Keto?

The primary focus of the keto diet is to incorporate more fats and fewer carbohydrates. The diet is built around activating ketosis, a process within your body where fats are burned for energy due to a lack of carbs. The ketosis process is meant to imitate fasting, so it works to use up energy sources already stored in the body. By carefully choosing what foods you incorporate into your diet, you can have your body working overtime to shed the extra fat without starving yourself.

When you hit that ketosis sweet spot, it changes your metabolism and even gives it a little push. It also has the additional benefit of reducing that loud, nonstop appetite that ravages us in moments of weakness. It does this by decreasing the production of hunger-stimulating hormones and by feeding you filling foods. The proof is in the pudding: In 2013, a statistical study using randomized controlled trials following 13 people demonstrated how those who followed the ketogenic diet lost 2 pounds more than those on low-fat diets in a year (Bueno et al., 2013). Similarly, another review of studies followed 11 people over 6 months, and this study denoted how those who followed ketogenic diets lost 5 pounds more than their fad-diet counterparts (Mansoor et al., 2016). The best part about the keto diet is that you won't get those cravings you would have if following a low-calorie, no-food diet, because you'll be well fed.

Another way to think about the keto diet is that it aims to remove unnecessary ingredients, namely sugar and preservatives, from your daily intake. The problem with modern preservatives is that they can be found in almost every product you buy from your local store and are part of your monthly groceries, rippling from large corporations into your humble abode. The problem with this is that those additives are difficult for our body to digest and can sometimes lead to serious stomach-related diseases and illnesses. The keto diet advocates for using raw ingredients as much as possible to remove unnecessary harmful preservatives or additives. A rule I keep in my belt is to never eat anything you can't pronounce. You have to become healthy before you can start losing weight, and, to do so, you have to reset your body and train it from scratch.

When discussing the keto diet, it is necessary to address some common misconceptions, namely, that the diet is too strict and limited in taste. The keto diet utilizes foods that have been around for centuries and welcomes all variations. Plenty of greens, grains, superfoods, meats, and spices are allowed through keto, providing plenty of flavors. Many companies are now developing popular foods designed to be keto-friendly. In the *Big to Small* keto plan, many spices and flavor-packed foods are allowed, and it even contains a cheat day at the two-week mark. That's only two weeks out of a whole fifty-two weeks. There are few reasons anyone should feel restricted or bored with their meals on this plan.

Another misconception about the keto diet is that you must continue practicing the diet forever to lose weight. Many diets require complete lifestyle changes for extended periods of time or forever. While consistency is vital, through personal experience, we can guarantee that you can go off the diet and keep the weight off. Success is obtainable in a short, three-week span of time and through manageable, time-efficient workouts. I suggest a minimum one-week break between keto diet cycles.

You could also start looking into adding intermittent fasting techniques into your diet. Whenever you eat, your body releases insulin. The majority of the population has more insulin pulsing through their bodies than they need, and it is missed because most doctors only look at blood glucose and blood pressure. The goal of this is to lessen the amount of times that you eat without decreasing the amount of calories that you're consuming. I suggest going three meals without snacks and then going two meals and maintaining that. It resets your body by helping it retain nutrients better because it will be storing them and using them more efficiently. This does not mean that your body will hold onto all of the food you're eating but instead just the nutrients.

This means your body will become more adept at saving and supplying your body to meet all its needs. So, if you'd like to try this alongside your keto journey, then go right ahead!

Chapter 1: Getting Started

Congratulations! You are taking the first important step. There is quite a bit of information to go over, but, as with all outstanding accomplishments, take it one step at a time. To start the keto diet, you must understand the best practices to follow and some habits to avoid.

For your success, do what you know will work for you. Understanding your body and your cravings is important when taking advantage of the keto diet. We only crave foods because your body is used to a routine or certain source of energy. Whether it be the power-pushing sugar or consistent cups of coffee to push you through the day, that's why you should know your weaknesses—for me, it would be the late night snacks.

The keto diet is intended to cleanse your body of unhealthy and processed foods. Do not set unrealistic goals that will cause you to fail, which I know you won't. The benefit of this plan is that it's made to be repeated and reused. Start with small, achievable goals to familiarize your mind and body with the changes. If you find a particular milestone hard to achieve, work on completing just that one for the duration of the 21 days.

Another key to success is dragging some friends or family along with you. Devise a great way to compete with those around you, and push and support each other to achieve your goals. As they say, it takes a nation and strength only the determined possess. If you do not have this, simply have someone you can talk to about the diet. There are also plenty of social media groups to share your journey. Collaborate with others on a similar path, and learn from those around you. Letting at least one other person know and having them check in with you is a great way to decrease setbacks.

The last major essential part of the keto diet is consistency. You will find the first few days will test your willpower, but you have the power to push through. It is easy to fold when hunger overwhelms inspiration, or your schedule doesn't allow time to cook healthier meals. While it is acceptable to have to restart the diet if you fall off the wagon, try your best to stay focused and satisfied. The only thing that works is planning! Think about the times you may have failed a diet before. What situation or feeling contributed to that? Now, make a plan to avoid those previously detrimental situations. Knowing your triggers will help you avoid them and stay the course.

Ready, Set, Goal!

Just as a professional athlete must strategically adjust their plan to score, you must do the same to achieve your goals. A well-thought-out goal will challenge you to push yourself and manage to achieve it. There are plenty of methods for setting a goal, but a highly-recommended one is S.M.A.R.T. goals; the simplest way to explain it is to expand the acronym.

S—Specific

Being *specific* is the first step, and by focusing on your keto diet, you have already completed the first step. A goal without a particular outcome in mind complicates the rest of the planning. You must know what outcome you want in order to decide how to achieve it. Specificity is easily achievable because you know what to do. So, take advantage of the advice given and you've got it under wraps.

M—Measurable

A *measurable* goal has steps you can track and milestones you can achieve. There needs to be a part of the goal where you can track your progress. For example, the keto diet may look like losing weight or incorporating healthier ingredients into your diet over time, but you could also use that journal I mentioned earlier. Humans are very visual creatures, and that is why using pie charts or graphs is easier for us to comprehend or accept.

A—Attainable

The *attainable* piece of the planning requires you to set a goal you can honestly complete. This step requires the most foresight because you have to be introspective and know your weaknesses. Think about roadblocks, personal habits, and time. The amount of support from others in your life, temptation, and unpredictable life events are all great examples of obstacles that could prevent you from completing the diet. Additionally, think of your habits and keep them in mind constantly. Maybe you eat midnight snacks, have a glass of wine when you get stressed, or always go out to eat for dinners on Saturdays; identify those behaviors that may be second nature to you now but could derail your progress. The last piece of advice is timing out your diet. Take into account when holidays are and which holidays are related to feasts. Also, simply think about your daily schedule and how you will need to fit in exercise, cooking, and meals.

R—Relevant

The *relevant* piece of goal setting is meant to keep the plan focused on the short- and long-term goals. For example, on the keto diet, you may have to try new foods to keep the meals interesting. While it's helpful to try new ingredients, making that a goal of your diet plan would distract from the overall goal which is to lose weight. Keep your short-term goals cohesive with the primary end goal. So basically, you should fake it until you make it.

An additional piece to relevant goals is to make sure that they are goals aligned with your thoughts and beliefs. You will fail if you do not believe in the plan you created.

T—Time Based

A good goal will challenge you to make necessary changes by a specific date. When determining the *time* length, you need to allow an adequate amount of time to reach your milestone. It will not be possible to drop a lot of weight in smaller time frames; instead, put reasonable due dates on losing smaller amounts of weight. For this particular plan, the time frame is set for you. But, remember to be honest with yourself and readjust the schedule as needed.

The Big to Small Keto Diet Plan

There are a few pieces that come together to create the whole picture of this version of the keto diet. Beyond just what you portion for yourself each day, there are specific foods and drinks you can or cannot have. The plan below will be the suggested starting point but is not meant to be the only way you can go keto. Cater the program to your needs, but understand the same results cannot be guaranteed.

This diet will last for three weeks. During this time, you will need to eat at least three meals and two snacks per day while consuming the suggested daily water intake. Focus your diet on consuming more healthy fats than protein or carbs in each meal and snack. We will not tell you exactly what to eat or how much because that will depend on your lifestyle and activity levels. For example, someone with lots of physical activity in their day will need more food than someone with a more sedentary lifestyle. The only limitation suggested is the number of meals with carbs. The first week allows for four meals, the second week allows for three, and the last week will ask you to only have two meals with carbs.

While correctly portioning your diet, there are a few foods and drinks you should not consume. First, the consumption of alcohol is not allowed while on this plan. There are no valuable nutritional ingredients in alcoholic beverages, and they will only work to slow weight loss. Second on our list are processed foods. This refers to most grocery items in jars, containers, or packages. Most processed foods are high in sugars, carbs, and fats that will work against the purpose of this diet. Lastly, anything with high amounts of sugar, or sugar at all, is not allowed; this also includes artificial sweeteners. Removing sugar from your diet will help you avoid most foods that are not keto-friendly. There will be sugar withdrawal if your body has grown addicted to it, so account for this when setting the parameters for your diet.

Exercise will work to burn through the body's fat stores as you consume energy. The minimum amount of suggested activity is thirty minutes for at least four of the seven days in the week. Since there are so many types of exercise, there is a dedicated chapter to suggested workouts. The type of exercise is up to you, but challenge yourself to do something that will get your body working. If you are not using up stored fat, the results will not be as beneficial to your goals.

When you have completed the initial thirteen days of the diet, you are allowed one cheat day. On this day, you are welcome to eat and drink whatever you would like, but then you'll fast the following day. The day of fasting will include only consuming your drinks for the day, such as water and green tea. Please proceed with caution when fasting. If you have any preexisting medical conditions that could cause health concerns, please eat smaller portions that following day. We intend to rid your body of the excess nutrients, not deprive it of them or endanger it.

In the last week of the diet, remember you're asked to limit your carbs to only two of your meals. Finish out strong! If it's difficult to return from the cheat day, find new recipes or ingredients to keep you interested. In the end, weigh yourself, and then reflect on what you have put yourself through and what you may change next time. Here are a few questions to help you start:

- How do you feel physically and mentally compared to three weeks ago and now?

- What were your energy levels like through the diet?

- Did you notice any changes after cleansing your body from sugars and processed foods?

- How did your cheat day make you feel?

- What foods did you find that you now love?

- How much weight were you able to shed?

If you have achieved the result you were looking for, congratulations! If you want to see more changes, we suggest allowing a minimum of a week's break. While in between diet cycles, still try to incorporate some new recipes you learned or keep your sugar and processed foods intake down. You do not want to diminish all the hard work you just put in.

Keto S.M.A.R.T. Goal

Now, let's put the previously discussed S.M.A.R.T. goal method and go over the suggested keto plan.

S—Specific

The diet is specifically the keto diet. It requires balancing the nutrients in each meal, snack, and drink. Specifically, your meals will involve protein, vegetables, and a small portion of carbs. The recommended carb intake changes with each week you continue the diet. There will also be snacks throughout the day that usually call for fruit and protein in the form of nuts. You cannot consume alcohol or sugary drinks.

What do you want to accomplish? There are many benefits of doing the keto diet, any of which should help keep you motivated and help specify what changes you would like to see. Change is the best motivator, especially if it's a good change. The most obvious reason to complete the keto is to lose weight, and it's a great way to reset your body to keep the weight off.

There's nothing worse than having to deal with a prepubescent nightmare as an adult. If you're suffering with acne, just remember that 3 in 4 people from ages 11 to 30 are dealing with the same issues. So, if you're struggling with adult acne, then doing the keto diet is a great way to clear it up; a great skin care routine wouldn't hurt alongside the diet. Interestingly enough, there are many causes of acne, but one cause seems to have links to diet and blood sugar in some people. So, if you are currently eating a diet high in processed and refined carbohydrates, you might be affecting the bacteria in your gut that cause your blood sugar to rise and fall significantly. Your skin is not a huge fan of change, and it only reacts with acne to let you know that something is wrong. One skin necessity you should keep on your toiletry shelf is tea tree oil. It's great for healing scars and evening your skin tone, and you can use it on any scars or even stretch marks. One thing you should keep on your kitchen counter is tea. A cup or two of black tea per day can change your skin forever. The polyphenols in tea reduce sebum production which could calm down the acne. It is better to have it in a topical form, but starting a habit of drinking tea is extremely beneficial for your skin.

There are even some researchers out there that have pursued their interest in the keto diet into its possible effects on cancer. A question was raised about the diet's effect on our cells and how they change their function in relation to how they might affect cancer cells. Cancer cells change metabolism functions by increasing tumor-growing cells. This is a natural process in humans, but cancer cells increase glucose and hydroperoxide metabolism which are supposed to compensate for those increased tumor forming species. This means that cancer cells feed off of glucose to stop these tumor-causing species, but by doing so, they simultaneously increase in size themselves. So, the hypothesis arose that by diminishing glucose and carbohydrates and implementing a diet higher in fat, the cancer cells would have less to feed off from, and, thus, the healthy cells would do better as well. Therefore, by starving the cancer cells, treatments like chemotherapy have more of a chance to destroy the starved cells.

The *Big to Small* plan also affects the heart for the better, but you have to do it right. So, being prepared is also important in specifying your goals. The keto diet has shown its heart-saving powers through lowering bad cholesterol and raising good cholesterol. Even though the thought of eating fats sounds good, you have to distinguish between the good and the bad.

But wait, there's more for you to hold onto through the next two weeks. When your body is in a state of ketosis, there are ketones that are released which have a neuroprotective impact on aging brain cells. On top of this, they also have anti-inflammatory properties and increase the function of our cells through the powerhouse of the mitochondria. They do this in much the same way as starving the cancer cells, but, in this case, we focus on the power-boosting effects on our healthy cells and brain cells as well. What might interest you further is that our brain is the only organ that can use ketones in place of glucose at a sufficient level for it to survive.

That covers some points to answer why you're doing this. Next, you should ask why these goals are important. Of course we would all love to be a little lighter and experience fewer symptoms of an unhealthy diet. But why not look into achieving it to prove that you can? This is one of my best motivators because I love finishing something I started: "Starting strong is good. Finishing strong is epic" (Sharma, n.d., para. 1). Simple quotes will change your day, and repeating a mantra will make your subconscious remember it. Visualizing your success is what's so important about this first phase. Be specific, envision your success, and imagine yourself as having accomplished this feat; your mind is half the battle.

Then, you should ask about who's involved. You are, of course, but who else is alongside you? Often, thinking about living longer and getting to spend more time with my family and friends leaves me feeling empowered and purposeful. This diet expands far beyond what you put in your body and what you don't. It's a tool you can use to change your everyday life and your life 10 years from now. But, the later you start, the longer you'll wait.

The next question is quite an easy one to answer: Where is it located? The answer would be everywhere because food is constant. The goal here is to exclude those locations that make it hard to stick to the plan. Don't avoid living life, but maybe try some different activities that are physical. There's a lot to do out there: You could visit a park for an afternoon picnic under the trees, go bird watching, or enjoy a scenic hike with the fresh air and flowering flora. One of my favorite activities is simply going out and finding new activities. Luckily, in the 21st century, we have wonderful technology that shows us what's in the area, what's free, and what's active. Give it a try and maybe find a new hobby.

Lastly, decide on what resources are limited. If you don't have a lot of time for meal prep, then look into doing a do-all-Sunday. Make Sunday morning prep time, and think about what meals you're going to do throughout the week. This seems a bit tedious, but it is why specific is a part of the S.M.A.R.T. goal plan. Afterwards, make a trip to the local shop and grab all your ingredients. Try the diet domino which means that you'll use yesterday's leftovers today, especially if you leave early for work in the mornings. You could even pack it up the night before and grab it on the go. It's better and cheaper than stopping at a fast-food chain in the middle of the day during traffic in your one-hour break. If you stay at home or work from home, then you may also do this to avoid doing the dishes or thinking about what to make.

M—Measurable

Your success with the keto diet will be measured by the continual, day-to-day fulfillment of the requirements. Additionally, the daily weigh-ins will help you track your weight loss progress. But there's a lot more to measure than just the weight loss. The best part about the measurable step is that it's useful when planning ahead. Set small measurable goals like how much water you're drinking and how often you stick to your new workout regimes, even if it's a daily evening, 15-minute walk. A measurable 15 minutes could make the world of difference mentally. It also makes dinner more delicious, so think about how much, how many, and by when you'll hit your target. These questions are important because breaking things down into smaller goals that are easier to achieve is important for morale and self-persuasion.

So, how much do you want from this diet? The answer is simple: It's how much you want to put into it. Consider the example of filling up your piggy bank: If you don't put any money into it, you're losing money when you break it open because you had to buy it. If you're buying all the ingredients and paying for all the extras without putting in the time or determination, then you're already starting at a deficit. How many days are you planning on staying on the diet, and which days will you take off? This diet does allow a cheat day, and I can promise you that your cheat day is far more rewarding if you make the most of the days when you're on the diet. The hardest part, though, is that day after cheat day. You have to push through it and keep yourself busy so you don't have time to reminisce about the delicacies the day prior. Lastly, how will you know when it's done? Keep that last day in mind when making any decisions, because, if you do the *Big to Small* method right, that day will be revitalizing.

A—Attainable

Even if you build your diet on the foundation outlined, you can manipulate it however you desire to make it fit your lifestyle. The keto diet is possible for anyone because you can cater it specifically to yourself. The diet provides nutrition for survival and daily function as well as supports your overall health.

I know that you can do it. Attitude is 90% of the battle, and keeping yourself in the zone is attainable. This step also involves what you've specified. Nothing is done without a little willpower, and there are countless techniques out there to help you achieve these goals. S.M.A.R.T is one of the best ones to use. But, looking at the constant desire to do something is an ugly beast, and the best thing you can do is surround yourself with other people who enjoy achieving things. Their success will show you that nothing is impossible. Something I like to do is set goals alongside rewards. Now, whatever your reward may be, it must be attainable and something that will keep pushing you. For me, a reward would be doing something nice for myself. Whether it be going for a massage or cheating on one of my workouts by watching a film I've been wanting to see for a while. Small changes can really make a world of difference. Avoid burning yourself out; that's why most people fail because they go too hard too quickly. Take your time because you have a lot of it. If you're having a hard day, call someone or vent your frustrations. Be easy on yourself because everyone falls short sometimes, but you have to get back up and keep fighting. My secret weapon is watching and listening to motivational speeches or finding some helpful tips and tools from people I admire and look up to, because they can give you mental strength through their words and actions.

R—Relevant

Each part of the plan is meant to work together. The focus on high, natural fats will replace carbohydrates. As you exercise, your body is using up stored carbs—which are in low supply now—and then burning fat to maintain its energy levels. These combined changes in diet and activity levels will ensure weight loss.

So, when looking at the relevance of changing your life for a couple weeks, you should ask yourself a couple of questions and answer them as best you can before you start. Ask whether it's worthwhile for you to go on this journey. Of course, you want to lose weight, but are you going to stick to the diet to achieve the results you want? Is it the right time for you to have to pay attention to your diet and every meal you're going to be eating? Will you be able to accomplish all of the required steps in order to complete the challenge?

These questions are difficult because we're never truly prepared for life, but I suggest planning it a week after a holiday. You'll already feel prepared to not eat all of the delicious holiday junk foods. You'll also be in a routine because of work, and this starting point gives you a breather before jumping into a different lifestyle for a couple of weeks. Therefore, during that first weekend back at work, you should sit down and understand this book; you will need to think about budget, prep days and materials, weekly goals, and have a look at the S.M.A.R.T method of doing things. Then, I would suggest saving your cheat day planning for a free day because it will give you some perspective of time and goals.

Also, look into whether it fits into your other priorities or commitments. If you know there's a lot of birthdays around the corner or a lot of family events, then it might not be the right time. With that being said, it might never be the right time and there will always be unexpected hurdles, but a little forethought goes a long way into succeeding. You might also need to look at your expenditures and payments throughout the month; knowing how much you have to spend on the diet is helpful when planning meals.

T—Time Based

The diet is set on a strict, three-week schedule each time you complete it. The daily planning of meals is spaced out to allow snacks to reduce hunger pains. Your cheat day is placed two-thirds of the way through. This keto diet plan is strategically mapped out daily, guaranteeing your progress and weight loss.

Baby steps are the way to go. What can you do today? What can you do this week? What can you do in the next six weeks? These questions are helpful when you're in the dumps, because just thinking about what you can do in the next minute or hour could mark the difference between breaking your bond with your diet—and feeling horrible for a couple of days—and a moment of strength for a week of joy.

Chapter 2: Consciously Consume

When you limit what you utilize in meals, it challenges you to be aware of what you put in your body. Since the keto diet works by incorporating naturally grown foods that have been around for hundreds of years, the meal possibilities are endless since they consist of century-long catalogs of recipes. Pay attention to how your body reacts to different foods, and notice how a few ingredients can go a long way with the proper seasoning.

Nutrients go beyond what you put in your mouth. The correlation of foods we ingest includes the physical results of either poor or healthy dieting. The saying that abs are made in the kitchen not at the gym is relevant throughout your entire journey to weight loss. Try to find peace in the space where you make your meals. While cooking, try to focus on how that food is influencing your life, and remember that the time you put into making meals will culminate into tangible results that you'll see after the keto process is complete.

Your body will go into a state of total redemption. You'll drop in weight and gain muscle, and you'll notice a change in your metabolic processes afterwards. Astoundingly, it has been used to treat epilepsy and obesity since the 1920's (Allen et al., 2014). Recently, its powerful effects have been tested on pathological conditions like acne, polycystic ovary syndrome, diabetes, neurological diseases, cancer, and it indicates improvement in respiratory and cardiovascular disease risk factors (Paoli et al., 2013). Therapeutic disease research done with the ketosis process shows the effect of this diet on the diseases and illnesses mentioned above.

One of the best reasons to begin this diet and consume consciously would be the respite from stress for your country's health system. By using your diet to avoid these diseases and ailments, you could change the world for those who can't afford appropriate hospital care.

What Can I Eat?

What can you eat? is the million dollar question. Before you think about the things you can't eat, think about why you can't eat them. You and I both know they're tempting, but what if I told you that you don't really enjoy them? This is due to the bacteria in our gut that communicate to our brain that they want high-fat, high-sugar foods because it's a quick source of energy.

Whatever you do, don't go back to oily, fatty foods when you've completed this diet. Yes, they're delicious and most would agree with you. But, they are also well hidden, extremely addictive, and disastrously dangerous. They can be found in sugary drinks, hamburgers, fries, packet chips, doughnuts and other baked goods, margarine, coffee creamers, sweet treats, packet microwave popcorn, fried mozzarella sticks, and all those other "good" foods. What they all have in common is that they have been chemically altered and, therefore, are harder to be understood or digested by your body. The main issue with low-density lipoproteins is that they can't be digested by your liver and removed from the body, so they tend to float around in your arteries until they settle somewhere in the bloodstream and block blood from smoothly pumping through.

As mentioned previously, the keto diet requires high-fat, moderate-protein, and low-carb food intake. There will be moderation and balance, but the essential changes from a typical diet will be in those three areas. Don't forget your fruits and veggies; they should be incorporated into daily meals as usual. If you're still questioning how many is enough, then twenty to thirty different kinds per week is a suitable amount to follow. You should try to keep them as diverse as possible; there are endless amounts of plants and trees out there, each with individual fruits, leaves, or even whole heads, all of which carry added benefits. By keeping your fruit and vegetable intake varied, you can change a lot more than just your weight.

While there are plenty of suggestions, you don't need to limit yourself to what's only mentioned in this book. Each person differs from the next, so keep in mind that trying various combinations will make it easier for you to succeed on this journey. Your primary focus should be setting a realistic balance for your lifestyle. For example, someone working in an office most of the day will require fewer carb-heavy items than a professional trainer working out with clients all day. Some items high in necessary carbs will fit into their diet but not yours. Fear not, as there will be more than enough to start you off and keep you going through your journey.

Much of the fats we encounter today come from processed foods, or foods that have been changed from their natural state. While, at its core, processing food can be as simple as heating it up, the harmful bits we should actually care about are those with too many added ingredients. It can also be said that almost every meal you get from a restaurant or make at home has carbohydrates in them. Recall that ketosis means your body is low on glucose—which carbohydrates and processed foods are rich in—and that when you restrict carbs and glucose, your body has to look elsewhere for energy, meaning it turns to ketones found in your food as well as to body fat. The cool thing about this diet is that you don't actually have to starve yourself. Much like any other diet, calories are restricted, prompting the body to turn to other sources of fuel and begin weight loss. The difference between *Big to Small* and other fad diets is that you're tricking your body into thinking you're starving but pulling a fast one by eating plenty of the right foods.

A good tip for knowing where the processed foods are is to look at a grocery store and how it's laid out. Keeping to the outer walls will keep your choices keto-friendly; that's where you'll find fruits, vegetables, meats, and healthy fats like dairy. Most items purchased in the center aisles of the store should be avoided except for grains or cooking oil. If you can find a farm-to-table situation, you can carry this deal through the rest of your life.

Fats

The keto diet is easily distinguished from others by its praise of fats, but that doesn't mean fatty foods. It'd be all good and well to gorge onto a nice, greasy, dripping burger, but it won't do any good here. There are saturated and unsaturated fats, and they're the opposite to one another. The diet looks to get you turning your diet into 80% fat which is the optimal amount to force your body into ketosis. Remember that if something contains saturated fat, it's not good for you. If it's unsaturated, then it's good to go on that diet. It also improves your insulin sensitivity which can aid your weight in the long term.

Fat has been a part of the human diet since it began. If you wanted to get into the scientific details, you'll find that fat was beneficial for hunter-gatherer societies because it allowed for extended energy between meals. The need for drawn out energy stores is not as crucial today since we have 24-7 access to food. While our minds understand grocery stores and fast food, our bodies are still programmed to like fatty foods and store energy. Our muscles respond better to unsaturated fats, and it will be easier to put on muscle mass if you're on the keto diet.

Here are some of the keto diet-approved fats.

Nuts and Nut butter

Nuts are a superfood and can be a great addition to any diet. There are so many amazing facts about nuts as well as so many different kinds. In fact, ½ cup of mixed nuts provides you with a whopping 13 grams of protein. There are more reasons for this food type's classification as a superfood. They're crammed with minerals, fiber, healthy fats, and antioxidants.

Walnuts are chock-full of vitamin E which is good for the heart. More than that, it's rich in minerals like iron, manganese, phosphorus, calcium, and copper. It's great, but what does that mean for you? If you just add 3 ounces of walnuts to your daily diet, you'll experience numerous health changes for the better. In fact, here are four ways that walnuts can benefit your health.

Firstly, a study done at Pennsylvania State University found that if you replace your saturated snacks with unsaturated walnuts, you'll improve your blood pressure and experience other heart health benefits (Tindall et al., 2019a). The composition of walnuts contains certain compounds that feed the good bacteria in our gut, which means that you could experience less inflammation in your gut. This is because it protects the lining of your gut wall and might also help with any constipation or diarrhea.

Secondly, walnuts also show changes with a bacteria that has a lot to do with the regulation of blood pressure, suggesting a lowered risk of heart problems. This is due to the phytosterols which are a preferred cholesterol for your body, meaning there's less of a chance of your body absorbing other kinds of cholesterol.

Thirdly, walnuts contain polyphenols, also known as ellagitannins, which turn to urolithins after being metabolized. Urolithins are compounds that have antioxidant, anticancer, prebiotic, and anti-inflammatory properties. The other obvious benefit is the effect of phytosterols found from walnuts upon our cholesterol. Chowing down on this plant compound lowers your total cholesterol by 10% and your bad cholesterol by up to 14%. The National Education Program implores those with high cholesterol to consume at least 0.1 ounces of phytosterols a day (Cohut, 2020). They are present in most nuts and some vegetable oils.

Lastly, they'll help you improve your mood and might even help you sleep. Walnuts are a wonderful source of phytomelatonin. What's quite mind-bending, and often overlooked in today's busy society, is the multi-faceted function of melatonin. It's naturally produced in your pineal gland and has anti-obesity, antioxidant, anti-inflammatory, and even anticancer effects; it even has neuroprotective attributes and effects. Therefore, it is undoubtedly one of the most important chemicals you should consume.

In combination with the effects from walnuts, you should also try to focus on putting those devices away as soon as it starts getting dark. Your brain knows to produce melatonin when the night takes over the day. You've been programmed like this since the beginning of time and for good reason. When the light begins to fade, your pineal glands release melatonin, and your body proceeds into a natural circadian rhythm. When you're all sleepy and ready for bed, you lay down and drift off into the first phase of sleep. The next stage is when your brain waves slow down, causing your heart rate and breathing to slow down as well. After this phase, the deep sleep and the brain activity that follow are known as delta waves. These brain waves are critical to restoring your body as well as your mind. In this phase, your brain analyzes all of your thoughts, experiences, and memories from that day and processes them. During the delta wave phase, your body releases growth hormones to repair muscle tissue, regrow bone cells, and strengthen the immune system. Then, we hit our rapid eye movement (REM) sleep cycle which is the most well-known phase of sleep, and our brains are almost as active as when we are awake during this phase. There's evidence that REM sleep impacts insightful thinking, creativity, and memory. What's interesting about this is that this is also when we dream, but these dreams are so much more than just a random series of events; it's more of a hard-drive clean up because it rids the brain of any irrelevant or unnecessary information. So, after seeing how important this mechanism is, think about how detrimental to your health using devices after dark can be.

Another common nut is the *pecan*, and it too has its place within the keto diet. Pecans are high in fat and are literally almost the same weight in fat as they are in grams. They also influence our insulin levels, a fact confirmed when two groups of middle-aged, obese patients were placed on two seperate diets. One diet was pecan-rich, and the other was basically the generic form of the pecan-rich diet. The generic diet consisted of the same amount of fat and fiber as the walnut diet, but the diet was nut-free. The results showed that there were significant beneficial changes in insulin resistance, regulation of insulin, and the function of insulin cells (McKay et al., 2018). They can also be used in many ways when cooking—I love to crust my fish or chicken in with pecans.

My personal favorites are those creamy *hazelnuts* that are rich in vitamin E; in only one serving, or 1 ounce, you get a banging 28% of your daily intake. This vitamin is great for the heart and is packed with antioxidants that fight off free radicals. Free radicals are basically cells in the body that are incomplete and, as such, are always looking for other cells to feed off from, but by doing this, they turn that cell into a free radical too. These guys usually end up creating tumors consisting of free radicals or the destruction of healthy cells. What's worrying about this is that there are no real symptoms of these buildups until serious illnesses arise.

The body produces antioxidants naturally, but the antioxidant production slows down as we age, so our body cannot effectively fight off free radicals the more we age. Therefore, being aware of adding antioxidants to your diet is a great idea. Hazelnuts also influence your cholesterol statistics. A study of 48 adults revealed that those who consumed an ounce of hazelnuts every day reduced their total cholesterol but increased high-density lipoproteins (HDLs), or good cholesterol, and vitamin E levels (Tey et al., 2010). In addition, hazelnuts are great as a sneaky treat in high-quality, dark chocolate bars.

What about *cashews*? They're a beloved nut because of their rich and creamy flavor, but they are also quite high in carbs with a net total of 8 grams per 1 ounce serving. Considering that your total daily carb intake is 2 ounces per day, cashews have a hefty control over what other carbohydrates you can add to the rest of your day.

While not commonly thought of as a source of fat, nuts are a favorite for the keto diet. They are suggested in many recipes and are also the main ingredient in your snacks. Most nuts are acceptable, with our favorites being macadamia or cashew; the same goes for butter. Avoid peanuts as much as possible as they lack the better nutrients found in other nuts. Most recipes can substitute butter with oil, but if you need butter, nut-based is better than most oil-based ones.

Coconut and Coconut Oil

Coconut oil is highly recommended due to its many benefits. Coconut is a "super metabolizer," meaning that it will work to speed up the metabolic processes in your body for hours after consumption. Coconut has a distinguishable taste that can add flavor but can also be suppressed with the right ingredients. It contains no sugar but offers a sweeter taste. For example, add a teaspoon of coconut oil to your coffee for flavor to notice the hint of sweetness.

With so many benefits, such as its high-lauric acid content, it's also known for reducing the release of the hunger-causing hormone known as ghrelin. Just think about the relaxing effect of quieting the "monster" within—the one that's screaming for doughnuts and bagels. Not only does it diminish your hunger hormone, it also boosts your HDL levels. We're all aware of good and bad cholesterol, but what is the difference? Well, it's quite simple really: HDLs consume cholesterol and transport it to your liver where it can be removed from your bloodstream, but low-density lipoproteins (LDLs) stay in your bloodstream and clog up your arteries.

The natural fat in coconut will help keep your fat intake higher with fewer foods to consume. Your body can also burn other fats because of the medium-chain triglycerides (MCTs) in coconut oil that are easily digested and immediately used for energy. It is a must to cook all meats, vegetables, and other foods with coconut oil. If you don't like coconut or are allergic, olive-based oils are the second-best choice. Try to find the purest coconut oil you can to avoid those preservatives or hidden fats. Finally, avoiding unnecessary, cheap additives in your coconut oil will increase energy levels and weight loss.

Avocado

Another superfood, avocado is an excellent source of fat. While technically a fruit, avocados work as a filling and comforting addition to almost any dish or as a snack on its own. There are over 20 varying nutrients in them, resulting in various benefits, including feeling fuller longer and aiding overall gut health. Not only are they delicious but they're packed with potassium. A total of 9 out of 10 Americans aren't getting enough potassium, yet the avocado is packed with 708 milligrams, or 0.02 ounces, compared to the measly 422 milligrams, or 0.01 ounces, in a banana. Plus, if you swap avocados for bananas, you can eliminate all that extra sugar. The avocado is also a good starter food for the keto newbie because it helps your body adapt to burning fat as fuel. It might also help fight off that "keto flu" because it boosts the keto adaptation process. A simple way to do this is by eating some salted avocados before meals, and you'll gain the added benefit of feeling fuller after eating.

Avocados contain a plethora of nutrients as well as a net-carb value of only 2 grams and 7 grams of fiber. They're packed full of vitamins, such as vitamin C, B5, B6, E, B6, B1, B2, and B3, and contain a sufficient amount of minerals like iron, zinc, copper, magnesium, manganese, phosphorus, and potassium. In addition, avocado oil has a very high smoke point, meaning that it doesn't oxidize as quickly as other oils. This is important because oxidized meat can be harmful to your health; it causes free radicals, especially through the charred bits.

Flax, Hemp, and Chia Seed

Consider these three the holy trinity of seeds that can be worked into many different types of dishes. *Flaxseed* has a flatter, bland taste and blends nicely into yogurt, smoothies, or overnight oats. Hemp has an earthy flavor and blends in well with vegetables or grains. Finally, chia seeds absorb a lot of water and work well in smoothies and yogurt. No matter which seed you add to your meal, all are rich in nutritious fats. Specifically, they all contain alpha-linolenic acid (ALA), an omega-3 fatty acid which is tied to improved heart health.

Individually, they offer unique nutrients. For example, flaxseed is rich in the B vitamin thiamine which is associated with improved metabolism. Be aware of the fact that whole flaxseeds are not digestible by your body. Avoid using them as they are; instead, break them down into a form your body can absorb all those nutrients from. You could try finding some milled or ground flaxseeds, or you could use a coffee grinder to achieve the same product. What makes them so desirable for the keto diet? They've actually been praised for years because of their properties. For one, they are packed with omega-3 fatty acids, lignans, and both soluble and insoluble fibers. Lignans are an interesting antioxidant because they have a plant estrogen that has shown positive effects on different types of cancer like colon and breast cancer. The soluble fiber of the flaxseed will help protect your heart and prevent diabetes. Both fiber types play a role in the digestive tract but also help with that hungry hormone "monster."

Hempseed is a good source of protein as well. Hemp is making a huge impact on the shelves. They have a lot of health benefits and are a great addition to the keto diet. In just 3 tablespoons of hempseed, you'll rack up a stocky 9.5 grams of protein. Just for reference, they have almost the same protein content as soybeans. They're also a complete source of protein which means they provide us with all 9 of the essential amino acids that our body does not produce. This is not a regular occurrence for plant-based proteins, which is why it's a great source of protein and fiber that provides us with a full feeling. To get enough fiber from your hempseed, try to find ones with the hull, or shell, on. It can also help stabilize your blood sugar, promote gut health, and help with weight management.

Two of the essential amino acids are omega-3 and omega-6 fatty acids. These fatty acids are extremely important for a healthy body and should be consumed with a balanced ratio between both types of fatty acids. A fascinating fact from an animal study in 2015 showed that hens that had hempseed and hemp oil added to their diet actually produced eggs with increased levels of omega-3 fatty acids in the yolks (Neijat et al., 2015). You should consume twice the amount of omega-3 fatty acids compared to other fats. Hempseed contains medicinal phytocannabinoids which have shown direct links to a system in our brain known as the endocannabinoid system (ECS) (Maroon & Bost, 2018). This setup has a hand in central nervous system development and homeostasis throughout the body. The ECS connects to every intersection of the body's multiple systems, allowing communication between all the cells. Cannabinoids even possess pain-relieving properties by calming the nerve cells at the site of injury, preventing excessive firing and even calming surrounding immune cells to stop the release of pro-inflammatory fighters.

Chia seeds are full of vitamins and minerals, such as calcium, iron, magnesium, and fiber, all of which work toward better gut health. As you can tell, you can't go wrong with adding these to any dish. They were extremely popular in the Aztec and Mayan civilizations because of their medicinal qualities. They were even used for religious rituals and cosmetics. These medicinal beliefs were actualized by modern science. Just 2 tablespoons of chia seeds contains 138 calories, 4.7 grams of protein, 8.7 grams of fat, 5 grams of ALA, 11.9 grams of carbs, 9.8 of fiber, 14% of your daily calcium, 12% of your daily iron, 12% zinc, and 15% of both vitamin B1 and B3. The antioxidants in chia seeds keep them from going rancid and benefit us as well. One of the most potent antioxidants is chlorogenic acid which feeds our GABA receptors and reduces our anxiety, lowers body fat by reducing triglycerides—which hardens your arteries—and bad cholesterol, prevents absorption and production of fats yet increases their breakdown simultaneously, improves cognition and memory, protects dopamine producing brain cells, and increases heart production and body fat loss.

Regularly eating chia seeds could also affect your bone health. Your bone mass begins decreasing after thirty, unless you're very active which helps them stay stronger for longer. Giving them an extra push is always a great idea. They assist in bone health because of their calcium, phosphorus, and magnesium content. We all know the importance of calcium and magnesium in bone health, but ALA might also play a big role in bone health. Studies have shown that it could improve mineral density which is crucial for bone strength and preservation (Lavado-Garcia et al., 2018).

Proteins

An essential part of any diet, proteins are great for building muscle, retaining muscle, and suppressing hunger. Protein is found in all types of food but is most common in meat. Since keto is focused on shedding fat and losing weight, protein's ability to retain muscle can become counterproductive to weight loss. Therefore, the *Big to Small* plan only allows protein in a select number of meals each week, so choose and ration wisely. Lastly, do not feel pressured to eat "super" meats. Make sure you buy what you'll eat; there are plenty of recipes out there that include your preferred proteins.

It might be common to hear that keto is meat heavy and that you'll be eating nice, juicy steaks, eggs, bacon, lettuce burgers, and tons of chicken breasts, but that's not all true. If you eat too much protein, your body begins a process called gluconeogenesis which produces glucose, and this will definitely kick you out of ketosis. The ideal ratio of macronutrients is 75% fat, 20% protein, and 5% carbohydrates. Therefore, only about ⅕ of your meal should be protein, so don't be looking for skinless chicken or an overdose of fish.

White Meat

Think along the line of birds and fish for this niche. Chicken, turkey, white fish, and salmon are all allowed on keto. Chicken and turkey are allowed as ground or minced, and turkey bacon is also allowed. Fish can be eaten in any form that meets the unprocessed and sugar-free restrictions. On this plan, light meat is only allowed for one meal during the week. Keep it fresh and keep it farmed is my motto.

Remember, you'll also want all that good fat in the skin on these meats, so include some nice juicy skin on chicken thighs and legs. Who doesn't love a good, juicy, roast drumstick? What's great about chicken is that you can roast it without extra oil if you do it right, so it stays juicy no matter what—I love using my air fryer for chicken wings especially on Friday nights. Also, look for skin-on fatty fish, because they're loaded with fatty acids and are just delicious overall.

Salmon is not the only keto-friendly fatty fish. Mackerel is a great fish to use, and so are sardines, anchovies, and char fish which are all delicious and nutrient rich. Some people might not feel so excited about sardines or anchovies, but they're flavorful and rich in nutrients. Anchovies, for example, are loaded with copper, a mineral that is hard to acquire from other foods. They also provide us with iron and an overwhelming amount of omega-3 fatty acids, actually more than the same weight of salmon. Anchovies also help us metabolize food into usable energy because of its vitamin B3 content. Its generous amount of selenium also boosts heart and thyroid function. Selenium has also been known to prevent the growth of tumors and fight off cancers.

Sardines are also a great addition to the keto diet because of their vitamin D content. They are also rich in B vitamins, especially B12 which is known as the energy and mood booster. Sardines also contain copper which plays numerous roles throughout our body, such as producing red blood cells, regulating heart rate and blood pressure, absorbing iron, activating your immune system, and production and maintenance of bones, connective tissue, and vital organs.

Some fish you should add fats to would be tuna, cod, seabass, and halibut.

Red Meat

Steak, hamburger patties, and pork are the familiar contenders in this category. Bacon is often associated with the keto diet, but our plan only allows thin-sliced bacon directly from a butcher. Additionally, the program only allows for red meats in two meals each week. Stick to fatty cuts of steak like the New York strip, rib eye, and brisket.

Egg

While not necessarily a category of its own, egg is a go-to protein choice while following this plan. You cannot beat this cheap, vitamin-rich, well-rounded protein. An egg has no restrictions on how many meals it can be utilized in, although you will still need to account for daily protein portioning.

Carbs

The enemy of most diets, carbohydrates are still essential to daily nutrition. Carbs are a building block for muscles throughout the body which has numerous benefits. Since it's excellent for building muscle, you will want to put your daily carb allowance in the meal closest to your workout. This does not mean eating a whole bowl of pasta but instead using "clean" carbs to maintain a healthy balance.

Sweet Potato

A well-known health food, sweet potatoes are an excellent fit for the keto diet. They have a taste that compliments or makes a great dessert or dish. Additionally, sweet potatoes can be utilized in many different shapes and consistencies.

Therefore, finding a way to use this superfood in a delicious recipe is not difficult.

Basmati Rice

Rice is a healthy carb, but basmati has less fat. For that reason, we suggest all rice be basmati. Also, since basmati has less built-in flavor than other healthy grains like jasmine rice, it's an adaptable part of any meal.

Gluten-Free Pasta

Gluten-free pasta has been compared to regular, gluten-filled pasta for years, but there is no additional benefit to weight loss. However, while no nutritional weight loss benefits exist, gluten-free pasta has fewer ingredients, meaning fewer additives in your diet.

Quinoa

Consider quinoa the secret agent of carbs. It's one of the only ones containing the same amino acids as proteins, meaning it has the nine necessary protein parts that our bodies need. As a result, quinoa will make a versatile, fulfilling addition to any meal.

Bran or Oats

Great additions to any smoothie or salad, bran and oats are great sources of healthy carbs. They make an excellent bed for any meat or vegetable and help you feel full. Perfect for any breakfast recipe, these two are sure to show up on your shopping list weekly.

Supplements and Spices

Not all necessary nutrients will be found in the foods and beverages allowed on the keto diet. To make up for the difference, take certain daily supplements to balance your health. Not all healthy foods have the best taste, so spice them up. Below, you'll find suggestions for both, but, as always, adjust the plan to yourself, your body, and your taste.

Vitamins

Vitamin C is a great addition to your daily diet. By putting more fruits and vegetables in your diet, vitamin C is naturally added to your system. On days when you find yourself eating less vitamin C-rich foods, take a tablet to keep your body's defenses up. According to the Mayo Clinic, vitamin C is great for keeping our internal systems balanced and fighting off diseases like the common cold in the short term and cancer in the long term.

Vitamin D will be a much-needed supplement during the keto diet. Since it's usually taken from foods like milk and fatty fish, which you're not allowed to have, it will be wise to keep vitamin D in your system. In addition, this essential vitamin strengthens bones and neurological functioning and reinforces your immune system. Don't pass by this one on the shelf, and be sure to add it to your daily intake.

Oils and Plants

Fish oil is a great way to obtain your omega-3 fatty acid without having to consume fish, and it's a perfect choice for those who don't eat it. Omega-3 fatty acids have many essential functions in the mind and body, such as muscle growth and function as well as cellular growth. Therefore, fish oil will provide essential nutrients for daily activities when taken in the correct dosage.

MCT oil may sound like a government experiment, but it's a superb oil packed with benefits. The oil has been studied and indicated a boost in energy and athletic performance and helped with making participants feel fuller. MCT will almost act like a replacement for the benefits of the sugars and carbs you no longer eat.

Dandelion root is a bit more of a personal choice. The plant has been found to have quite a few benefits in animals and humans. Dandelion helps flush out the body's system, so, in terms of weight loss, it will help shed some water weight. We suggest this additive more so in the last week of the diet, but feel free to dose it as it's healthy and beneficial.

Protein Powders

Protein powders will significantly benefit your diet since so many of your natural sources will decrease. How much protein powder you take will mostly depend on your exercise routine. I suggest whey protein since it's one you would have typically gotten from milk. In terms of the keto diet, whey protein powder is going to be a good muscle builder, and since it's in powder form, you can mix it with all types of foods, particularly in smoothies and shakes.

Spices

It cannot be stressed enough how essential spices will be in enhancing, changing, and creating new tastes and smells for your recipes. Your body will surely crave things you are now cutting out which will not be easy, but spices can help you recreate or invent new tastes. Additionally, spices are low in calories and keto-friendly, and they can replace some ingredients you may have sacrificed to keep your diet balanced.

Take a stroll down the seasoning aisle, and don't be afraid to try something. Find below a few favorites:

- *Chili* adds a smoky spice to any dish. It goes great on meats and vegetables.

- *Cinnamon* is a dupe for a sweet taste you can add to help wean yourself off sugar. Cinnamon can add a bit of sweetness to a meal or dessert, so enjoy finding the many ways you can work it into your diet.

- *Garlic* is one of the more iconic spices known for a very bold, robust flavor that makes a statement in any dish.

- *Onion* is the heart of flavor in many dishes, and it's no different when used as a spice. It will add a smell and taste of its own to bring the dish together.

- *Oregano* is known for a lighter taste with a peppery kick that will elevate the flavor of meats and vegetables. It's infamous in Italian and Latin cuisine, but oregano is versatile in almost any dish.

- *Paprika* is a great way to add a light spicy taste and enhance the flavor palette of your meals.

- *Pepper* is a must in almost any dish and will instantly add a smoky spice. There are very few recipes where pepper cannot fit in.

- *Red pepper flakes* are going to add some natural heat to your food. Add in a little bit or a lot, depending on your preference. This will alter or overpower the taste of whatever you use it on.

- *Rosemary* will blend well in savory, rich meats or vegetables to help round out salty or sweet tastes. In addition, it's known for pairing well with red meats.

- *Sage* has a similar role to rosemary but offers a strong, woodsy taste, so it will work best alongside other bold flavors.

- *Pink Himalayan salt* should be considered a built-in part of any recipe and takes the top spot for being the most useful. It will add a familiar, comforting taste to your dish, but be sure to use this in moderation to maintain a healthy balance in your daily sodium intake.

- *Thyme* is a spice that can do it all. It brings a savory and sweet taste, making it useful both in light and heavy dishes.

Chapter 3: Shopping Lists and Recipes

You may have noticed that the previous chapter included many food suggestions, each tying into a specific nutrient vital to the keto diet. Now, we're going to look at putting them together, mixing it up, adding a little here and there, and then enjoying a deliciously-seasoned, well-portioned, wholesome meal.

This might be your favorite part, and it's also the most motivating part of this whole process. We're adding to your old diet and making it awesome. There's nothing worse than scrolling through a ton of recipes only to find out you're missing one ingredient for each, and by the time you do, it's bedtime, and all you have the energy for is a sandwich. So, use the ones below that can be your tasty, trusty go-to's if you can't make up your mind. Shopping lists accompany them as well as a couple of staple foods that you can always have around to make a whole meal out of.

Time for Shopping

Grocery shopping for the right foods to avoid wasting can be overwhelming. This is because there are many variations of vegetables and fruits in produce alone. In contrast, if you walk down any aisle, you see how the packaging boasts how health-conscious it all is. We have a pro tip for keeping your shopping trips keto diet compatible. Try and stick to the outer edges of the store, and you will find yourself only shopping for produce, meats, and dairy. The only items you will need from the inner aisles will be oils and fat-dense products which are in limited supply with this diet and will be much easier to choose from. Joining a community or finding a local business that specializes in keto is a great idea as well. Spread your wings and use your feelers to find the best sources.

My advice would be to shop on the weekends. Try to purchase different things for each week. Since there are plenty of recipes later on in this book, I would suggest taking a peek at the recipes, write down the ingredients you need for the week, and then go grab your groceries. This is a 21-day lifestyle shift, so make it a fun 21. We are creatures of habit, but this also means that falling out of our everyday routine is difficult. We're also easily persuaded, so there's a fit for every fighter, and if you can figure it out, you're bound to win the fight.

Staple Foods

- Apples

- Frozen berries

- Oranges

- Pears

- Post-workout bananas

- Spinach

- Bell peppers

- Almond milk

- Green tea

- Lemons

- Full-fat greek yogurt

- Pink Himalayan salt

- Eggs

- Nuts—pecan and hazelnuts are my ultimate choices

- White meats

- Hempseed

- Chia seeds

- Coconut oil

Supplement Must-Haves

- Fish oil

- Vitamin C—1,000 mg daily

- Dandelion root—for the final week

- Magnesium—cramps, energy, immune function, and blood sugar levels

- Vitamin D—just good to have around in general

- Digestive enzymes

- Greens powder

Produce

Do not forget that vegetables and fruits also contain carbs which must be considered.

- Almond—whole nut, butter, flour, etc.

- Artichoke

- Arugula

- Asparagus

- Avocado

- Bananas—remember this is considered a sweet treat on keto

- Berries—blue, rasp, black, straw, etc.

- Broccoli

- Brussel sprouts

- Cabbage

- Cantaloupe

- Carrots

- Cashews
- Cauliflower—versatile
- Celery
- Cherry
- Coconut
- Cucumber
- Eggplant
- Grapes
- Green beans
- Hazelnuts
- Kale
- Kiwi
- Lemon—great for seasoning as well
- Lettuce—iceberg, romaine, etc.
- Lime
- Macadamia nuts
- Mango
- Mushroom
- Onion—red, yellow, Vidalia, etc.
- Orange

- Peach

- Pear

- Peas

- Peppers—jalapeno, bell, etc.

- Pineapple

- Pistachios

- Pumpkin

- Radish

- Spinach

- Squash—yellow, butternut, etc.

- Sweet potato

- Tomato

- Walnuts

- Watermelon

- Zucchini

Meat

Choose your meats wisely. Remember that certain meats are only allowed a certain number of times per week. Try to keep all meat skinless and as lean as possible.

- Chicken—breast, liver, thigh

- Turkey—ground, breast, leg, *bacon thinly sliced*

- Pork—chopped, steak, *bacon thinly sliced*

- Beef—ground, etc.

- Steak

- Fish—salmon, anchovies, sardines, tilapia, shrimp, etc.

- Egg

- Lamb

Dairy

- Milk—must be unsweetened; most nut-based milks will work

- Cheese—cottage, cream, sliced, shredded, cubed, etc.

- Heavy whipping cream

- Mayonnaise

- Yogurt—full-fat Greek yogurt is my favorite

Fats, Oils, and Others

- Avocado oil

- Butter

- Coconut oil—best

- Green tea bags

- Heavy cream

- Hot sauce—vinegar and water-based are best for avoiding unnecessary sugars and preservatives

- Olive and olive oil

Recipes

It would be unfair to bring you this far and not provide a few essential recipes to get you through the diet. These are a few recipes for meals, snacks, and drinks to get you thinking about others you may want to try. Ingredients and measurements will be based on one person's minimum daily intake, so please add and increase as needed.

A cool home trick would be to keep some easy flavor plants, or herbs, around. Grow some rosemary or spring onion on your kitchen counter, and grab a spring whenever you need it. There are all kinds of neat gardening setups these days. They've become easy, modern, sleek, and even centerpieces in some homes. Not only are they delicious, but they're also beautiful and add a lovely green tinge to your everyday life. All they really need is adequate sunlight, a little water here and there, nutritious soil that you can get almost anywhere these days, and a little trim every now and then.

A couple you could start off with are the ones that are staples in most flavor busters. *Parsley* is a great addition to the garden because it is one of the easiest to grow, mostly because it can be harvested at any time and pretty much just grows back by itself; you'll get a solid 12 months of parsley. You don't have to eat it all, but you could dry some for future use. It's best to plant them around autumn or spring, and keep them a little moister than other plants. In winter, they might need a little liquid fertilizer because they enjoy sunlight and moisture.

Mint is amazing because it's rather laid back. It doesn't mind the sun nor the shade and doesn't need much water, but it will spread like wildflower, so be sure to watch it's spread. It's better when you plant it in a container to mimic moist, dense soil. My favorite treat is the keto mint chocolate bar. It is the proverbial cliché to die for. In fact, my favorite sweet treat is a minty keto treat that is quite minty.

Before we get into the mouthwatering delight of these recipes, you have to remember that these should be used as a treat so as to not throw you off the trail. This is also great if you're just in the mood to bake something delicious especially for those small treat goals we spoke about.

Breakfasts

Because we're already placing our body into a state of ketosis, or fasting, the need for breakfast to break that fast isn't entirely relevant. But, eating first thing in the morning is great for your mood throughout the day; it helps with concentration and supports your body to regulate your weight as a result of consistent and regular replenishment. It also lowers your chances of eating cravings. When you're extremely hungry, your body craves juicy, greasy, and sugary foods which are to be avoided on the keto diet. If you're eating a tasty greek yogurt or another fermented dairy product along with other breakfast additions, then it could lower your risk of type 2 diabetes, cardiovascular disease, and inflammation, all of which is especially great if you're a gym freak.

Starting your day off right creates a precedent for the rest of your day, and that applies to your meals as well. Breakfast cannot, and will not, be overlooked while on the keto diet plan. There are infinite ways to create fulfilling, delicious meals that will get you started on the right foot at the start of your day. Many traditional breakfast dishes and drinks are compatible with keto, and here are a few to get you started.

Fully-Loaded Keto Breakfast Parfait

This is a quick breakfast that's easy to assemble. It's creamy, rich, and an absolutely juicy way to start the day. This is a great weekend treat or a Monday blues repellent. It's packed full of berries, nuts, cacao garnish, and coconut flakes. You'll love it if you're a fan of granola and missing your carb-filled granola fix. Here is the nutrition information for the keto breakfast parfait (Chef Sky Hanka, 2021):

Nutrition Facts
Breakfast Parfait

Amount Per Serving (4)	
Calories 340	

	% Daily Value*
Fat 33 g	42%
Carbohydrates 12 g	4%
Sugars 6 g	
Protein 14 g	
Vitamin A 2.11 mcg	
Vitamin C 3.07 mg	
*Percent Daily Values are based on a 2,000 calorie diet.	

What's in it:

- ½ cup heavy whipping cream

- 6 tbsp almond butter

- 2 tsp vanilla extract or some fresh ground vanilla pods

- ½ cup berries, such as strawberries, raspberries, or blueberries—my favorite is a strawberry raspberry mix

- 4 tbsp sliced pecans

- Fresh mint leaves for garnish and flavor

- Cacao powder for garnish

- ⅓ cup greek yogurt

Kitchen utensils needed:

- Mason jars or tupperware containers

- Measuring cups

- Tablespoons

- Spatula

- Mixing bowl

Right into the process:

1. Whisk together your yogurt, heavy cream, and vanilla into a mixing bowl. If you're looking to mix it up for this meal or the next time around, you could try adding some scrumptious dried spices.

   a. Pumpkin spice

   b. Nutmeg

   c. Lemon zest

   d. Ginger

   e. Almond extract

   f. Allspice

2. Line up your containers in a prep area. Spread out your yogurt delight into the jars at about halfway in

each container. Then, flatten it with your spatula—I like to use one of the rubber ones for a little extra give.

3. Grab your teaspoon, and place a decent dollop atop your flattened yogurt mix. I would suggest 1 ½ tablespoons in each, but how you lay it out is up to you.

4. Grab your berries, nuts, garnishes, and coconut flakes.

5. Place ⅛ of your chosen berries into each container. Sprinkle freely about to color it to your delight.

6. Topple in ¼ of the coconut flakes into each.

7. Drop in those beautiful brown pecans whole or chopped—it's up to you, but I like to just split them into halves or quarters.

8. Then, add another ¼ of your coconut flakes, making sure the mix is evenly spread.

9. Lastly, garnish with cacao powder and a sprig of mint.

You can keep the other containers in the fridge, and they should keep for a good seven days. So, there you go, no reason to skip breakfast if you've got backups in the fridge. You could also take one with you to work or scoff one down before a workout for a little sugar rush to push you through it. Here is the nutrition information for the breakfast mushroom and Parmesan cheese omelet (Pinney, 2017):

Mushroom and Parmesan Cheese Omelet

Nutrition Facts	
Mushroom and Parmesan Cheese Omelet	
Amount Per Serving (1)	
Calories 288	Calories from Fat 198
	% Daily Value*
Fat 22 g	34%
Carbohydrates 4 g	1%
Fiber 1 g	4%
Sugars 3 g	3%
Protein 20 g	40%
Vitamin A 830 IU	17%
Vitamin C 1 mg	1%
Calcium 281 mg	28%
Iron 2 mg	11%
*Percent Daily Values are based on a 2,000 calorie diet.	

Omelets will be a saving grace on the keto diet when it comes to staple foods that can change drastically in flavor. They are a quick fix for those who aren't keen on being up early before going about their day. You can mix and match proteins, vegetables, and spices to keep this classic dish feeling new each time around.

What's in it:

- 2 eggs

- Arugula

- 1 tbsp parmesan cheese—cubed or shredded

- ¼ cup sliced or diced mushroom of your choice—my personal favorite is the portobello

- A pinch of pink Himalayan salt

- A pinch of pepper

- A pinch of dried rosemary

- 1 tbsp water

- ½ tsp olive oil

- A sprinkle of the *Everything But the Bagel Sesame Seasoning Blend*

What's next:

1. Chop up those mushrooms whichever way you like, and put them in a pan with a little of that olive oil. Then, let them sit for about 3 minutes.

2. Crack the eggs into a mixing bowl, then pour a decent amount of water in to help fluff the eggs.

3. Next, you're going to want to heat your pan up—preferably nonstick to avoid added fats. Then, you're going to layer your pan with your salt, pepper, rosemary, and a little water to help the pan not stick, and follow up by spreading out all of your favorite flavors.

4. Pour those fluffy eggs into the pan, and let them sit.

5. To prevent the egg from burning or sticking to your pan, you can keep the omelet edges away from the pan. You can use a rubber spatula—it makes my life easier.

6. Layer your mushrooms onto the half-cooked, open omelet.

7. Place a couple of arugula leaves around the omelet.

8. Dust the omelet with the parmesan, and watch it melt.

9. Then, cover the pan for about 2 minutes.

10. Open it up, letting the steam free and the flavor escape. Grab and slide the spatula around one side of the omelet. Get really deep under there until about halfway and simply close the omelet.

11. Lastly, you can sprinkle a burst of flavor on the open omelet by adding the flavor acclaimed *Everything But the Bagel Sesame Seasoning Blend*. This thing is packed with flavor with its abundance of sea salt

flakes, sesame seeds, garlic, onion, and poppy seeds. It'll make that breakfast omelet a unique one.

12. Then, you can slip it onto your plate or into your lunch box. Open until it's cool or else it will sweat, and nobody likes sweaty eggs. You can even slip a piece of parsley on top to please the eye and be all fancy for breakfast.

Easy N'oat Bowl

This breakfast is oats without the oats. This is an all time favorite because I love those wholesome oats when they're a little sticky and chewy. You can add a wealthy topping of honey and a dollop of butter. Since you're adjusting for keto in this recipe, you might not include a big dollop of butter, but there will still be a lot of flavor. Here is the nutrition information for the n'oat bowl (Schiffer, 2016):

Nutrition Facts	
N'oat Bowl	
Amount Per Serving (1)	
Calories 453	
	% Daily Value*
Fat 36 g	
Carbohydrates 15 g	
Fiber 10 g	

Sugars 1 g	
Protein 18 g	
Vitamin A 155 IU	
Potassium 187 mg	
Calcium 165 mg	
Iron 6.5 mg	
*Percent Daily Values are based on a 2,000 calorie diet.	

What's in it—hint, not oats:

- ½ cup water
- A splash of your favorite kind of milk or cream
- 2 tbsp almond flour
- 1 tbsp chia seeds
- 1 tbsp golden flaxseed meal
- A small pinch of salt
- ½ tsp pure vanilla extract
- 2 tbsp hemp hearts
- 2 tbsp unsweetened shredded coconut

- Berries for sweetness—not included in the nutritional information

To the kitchen:

1. There's not much to it really; drop everything into a small pot over low heat.

2. Make sure it's constantly stirring for about 3–5 minutes.

3. Stir in the vanilla, and then eat it while it's still hot.

In the microwave:

1. This one is pretty much the same as before, but you'll drop in your water, almond flour, chia seeds, salt, hemp hearts, shredded coconut, golden flaxseed meal, and a pinch of salt.

2. Then, pop it into the microwave for 2 minutes until it's thick.

3. Lastly, stir in your vanilla, and it's ready to go.

I love this as a prepackaged lunch too, or even just a backup if I don't have time in the mornings. You can prepack a couple of the dry ingredients into containers or packets, and you'll have them ready to go whenever you want one.

Some variations:

If you're feeling extra spicy one day, then you can try out some of these different flavor combos.

Mango Madness

- Pop in ¼ teaspoon of ground cardamom while cooking.

- Then, scoop a lovely dollop of mango puree on the top or add some chopped mango.

Walnut Wonderland

- When the n'oat meal is cooked, you can drizzle 1 teaspoon of maple syrup over the steaming n'oats.

- Then, you can drop in 1 tablespoon of chopped walnuts.

Blueberry Blast

- After you've tipped your n'oats into your bowl, you can sprinkle in ¼ teaspoon of cinnamon.

- Then, pop in ⅓ cup of cooked or frozen blueberries.

Coconut Crunch

- For this one, you'll mix in ½ teaspoon of coconut sugar.

- Add in 1 slice of grass-fed butter.

- Then, you can sprinkle ½ teaspoon of cinnamon in there as well.

Popping Piña Colada

- This is one of my favorites! You'll top the n'oats with ⅓ cup of fresh pineapple.

- Then, add 1 tablespoon of shredded coconut.

Awesome Almond

- For a little nuttiness, add 1 tablespoon of chopped toasted almonds.

- Then, for the sweet part, add 1 tablespoon of dark chocolate chips.

- Lastly, top it off with 1 tablespoon of shredded coconut.

Strawberry Almond Cacao Smoothie

Smoothies will be a phenomenal resource for getting your necessary fruits and dairy in an addictive, on-the-go meal, or it can be a good meal if you don't love a heavy breakfast but know you should eat one. It's great because of its low-carb, high-fiber content. It contains more fat and protein than you'd think. Here is the nutrition information for the almond cacao smoothie (Tripkovic, 2020b):

Nutrition Facts	
Almond Cacao Smoothie	
Amount Per Serving (1)	
Calories 179	
	% Daily Value*
Fat 11.7 g	18%
Saturated Fat 4.3 g	22%

Carbohydrates 9.7 g	3%
Fiber 2.8 g	11%
Sugars 4.9 g	
Protein 10.7 g	
*Percent Daily Values are based on a 2,000 calorie diet.	

What's in it:

- ¾ cup strawberries

- 1 cup almond milk

- 2 tsp almond butter

- ⅕ scoop chocolate protein—my favorite is the *Kiss My Keto* brand

- 1 tbsp chia seeds

- 4 almonds

- ½ tsp vanilla extract

- 2 squares dark chocolate chopped, not chipped—you can also get this from *Kiss My Keto*

- Collagen

Ready, set, blend:

1. Lay out your ingredients—it's more satisfying that way.

2. Then, pop that blender lid and topple in the strawberries, almonds, chia seeds, almond milk, almond butter, collagen, and vanilla.

3. Close the lid—don't forget this important step—and blend it until it's smooth.

4. Slip it into a glass, then top it with your chocolate.

5. If you like the chocolaty bitterness of cacao, feel free to add some to the smoothie as well.

Summer Smoothie

This one's a bowl smoothie, and it's super low in sugar. Most smoothies get praise for being healthy and good for you, but most of them are filled to the brim with sugar and empty calories. This one is not, but it's a perfect summer breakfast treat or afternoon addition to lunch. It is quite high in carbohydrates but mostly fiber as well. It is also packed with avocado, so it will also keep your body full of healthy fats. Also, with a dash of lemon juice, the citric acid from the lemon will be good for that uric acid buildup. So, I highly suggest keeping these in rotation. Here is the nutrition information for the summer smoothie (Krampf, 2018):

Nutrition Facts
Summer Smoothie
Amount Per Serving (1 bowl)
Calories 319

	% Daily Value*
Fat 26 g	
Carbohydrates 15 g	
Fiber 10 g	
Sugars 2 g	
Protein 10 g	
*Percent Daily Values are based on a 2,000 calorie diet.	

What's in it:

- ½ scoop MCT oil

- 2 tbsp lemon juice

- ½ scoop collagen powder

- 3 tbsp sweetener

- ½ medium avocado

- ¾ cup coconut milk or any milk of your choice

- 1 cup spinach

- ¼ cup ice cubes

- ½ tsp chia seeds

- 1 tsp coconut flakes

- 1 tsp hemp seeds

What to do:

1. Grab the blender. Tip in the collagen powder, avocado, spinach, lemon juice, coconut milk, and the sweetener. Whir it up until it's green and creamy.

2. Pop the lid, and tip the ice in.

3. Blend until extremely smooth.

4. Pour it into your bowl of choice or in a takeaway cup, if you prefer.

5. Then, you can top the mix with the coconut flakes, chia seeds, and hempseed.

6. Enjoy!

Marvelous Muffins

I remember my favorite Sunday morning meal being warm muffins with melted butter and topped with cheese and jam. The way it all melted in your mouth was just heavenly. So, for me, these muffins were a godsend. These blueberry muffins will blow your mind and not the calorie count. Here is the nutrition information for the marvelous muffins (Laura, 2022):

Nutrition Facts
Marvelous Muffins
Amount Per Serving (1)
Calories 122

	% Daily Value*
Fat 10 g	
Carbohydrates 6 g	
Fiber 2 g	
Sugars 2 g	
Protein 5 g	
Vitamin D 1 mcg	
Potassium 35 mg	
Calcium 98 mg	
Iron 1 mg	
Vitamin C 10.3 mg	
*Percent Daily Values are based on a 2,000 calorie diet.	

What's in it:

- ¼ cup almond milk

- 1 tbsp coconut flour

- 1 cup almond flour

- 2 large eggs

- ¼ cup unsweetened almond milk

- ¼ cup sour cream

- ½ cup fresh or frozen berries

- ⅛ tsp salt

- ¼ cup allulose or erythritol for sweetener

- ½ tbsp baking powder

How to do it:

1. First, you'll want to pop your oven to 350 °F.

2. Slide over the mixing bowl, and mix together the dry ingredients: baking powder, salt, flour, and sweetener. On a side note, I've mixed these 2 flours mainly for texture, but if you'd like to use only a single flour, then I suggest 1 ¼ cups of almond flour.

3. Crack in the eggs and pour in the liquids: almond milk and sour cream.

4. Fold it all into each other, making sure to get rid of any lumps.

5. Pour the batter into the muffin tray.

6. Let them sit for 18 minutes.

7. You'll know they're ready when they're golden brown and the house is filled with a blueberry aroma. They should also not be spongy.

8. Note that if you're using frozen berries, let the muffins sit for 26–28 minutes.

Pop Tarts

These are great for your cheat day because they're quite the indulgence. Luckily, though, they won't make you feel as bad as real pop tarts! Also, it might be a fun family morning making some homemade pop tarts. Get the kids or just your significant other involved, and have a fun breakfast baking and making icing. Plus, you'll get some delicious, gluten-free pop tarts out of it. So, let's get popping, shall we? Here is the nutrition information for homemade pop tarts (Gore, 2021):

Nutrition Facts	
Pop Tarts	
Amount Per Serving (1)	
Calories 570	
	% Daily Value*
Fat 51 g	
Carbohydrates 46 g	
Fiber 7 g	
Sugars 4 g	
Protein 13 g	
*Percent Daily Values are based on a 2,000 calorie diet.	

What you're going to need:

- ¼ cup sugar-free jam

- 3 tbsp coconut flour

- ¼ tsp xanthan gum

- ¼ tsp kosher salt

- 1 large, beaten egg

- Egg wash

- ½ cup cubed cold butter

- ¼ tsp baking powder

- 1 tbsp Swerve Sweetener—granular

- Parchment paper

Glaze:

- ½ cup Swerve Sweetener—confectioners

- 1 tsp pure vanilla extract

- 2 tbsp and 1 tsp heavy cream

Let's make some tarts:

1. Make the crust first. Have your food processor or blender handy, or you could make it by hand.

2. Pop in the coconut or almond flour, sweetener, xanthan gum, baking powder, and salt. Mix it all together until it is evenly incorporated.

3. Then, add in your butter blocks. Either break up the butter into the mixture with your hands or pulse it in the food processor or blender.

4. Add your beaten egg, and then you can mix this in with a wooden spoon or pulse until it's all one delicious doughy mixture.

5. Plop the dough into a bowl, cover with a dish rag or plastic wrap, and refrigerate it for at least 2 hours.

6. While you're waiting, you can keep experimenting and planning out your meals for the week.

7. Place a piece of parchment paper on the counter. Gently flatten the dough so it's easier to roll. Place another piece of parchment over the dough, and roll it out into an 11-inch square about ¼ inch thick. If the dough cracks, just pinch it closed.

8. Slice the dough into 8 blocks that are each 2 inches wide and 5 inches long.

9. Spoon 1 tablespoon of jam onto 4 rectangles and spread it into an even layer. Leave a ½-inch border of space around the jam.

10. Place the other 4 pieces atop the jam.

11. Corrugate the edges of the tarts with a fork.

12. Preheat the oven to 350 °F.

13. Pop them in the freezer for 15 minutes.

14. Take them out of the freezer, and egg wash the squares generously. Then, bake them until they're

golden brown and their edges are firm. It should take 20–25 minutes.

15. While you're letting them cool, you can start on that glaze.

Glaze:

1. Grab your sweetener, heavy cream, and vanilla, and mix them into a small bowl.

2. Spread the mixture over the center of the cooled tarts.

Cereal Keto Lover

I love tossing this together and knowing I'll have a quick breakfast option whenever I need it. And, I love granola more than I should. One of my favorite breakfasts is a carby, sugary, granola-packed breakfast with all kinds of nuts and raisins, topped with a good helping of greek yogurt. This was a great keto option for me to swap out and curb those cravings, but be weary of your portion sizes. You could even sprinkle it over some keto ice cream; you can find the recipe under the Not So Sneaky Snacks collection.

Ingredients—3 cups:

- Cooking spray

- 1 cup chopped almonds

- ¼ cup melted coconut oil

- 2 tbsp chia seeds

- ¼ cup sesame seeds

- 1 cup chopped walnuts

- 2 tbsp ground flaxseeds

- 1 tsp pure vanilla extract

- ½ tsp ground clove

- 1 ½ tsp ground cinnamon

- ½ tsp kosher salt

- 1 large egg white

- 1 cup unsweetened coconut flakes

On a side note, you can swap out the almonds and walnuts for pistachios, pecans, or pumpkin seeds.

Get it going:

1. Preheat your oven to 350 °F, and grease a baking sheet with cooking spray.

2. Get out your large bowl and mix together the nuts and seeds plus the coconut flakes inside of it. Mix it well.

3. Pop in the cloves, cinnamon, vanilla, and salt, and stir.

4. Beat that egg white until it's frothy. Stir it into the granola mix.

5. Pour in the melted coconut oil, and turn the granola until it is all coated.

6. Spill the contents of the bowl onto the baking sheet, and spread with a spatula until the spread is even.

7. Let it stiffen and turn golden in the oven for 10 minutes.

8. Take it out, and give it a good mix. Pop it back into the oven for another 10–15 minutes.

9. When it's crispy, take it out and let it cool completely, or you could sneak in a bite.

Hearty Hash Browns

I am obsessed with eggs on hash browns, but on the keto diet, you can't stuff your face with those carby, oiled hash browns. So, I devised a plan to sneak them into your daily breakfast options. I heavily suggest these if you love a cooked breakfast.

What you will need—2 servings:

- ¼ small yellow onion

- 1 tbsp vegetable oil

- Freshly ground black pepper

- ½ tsp garlic powder

- 2 cups shredded cabbage

- ½ tsp kosher salt

Directions:

1. In a large bowl, you can whisk together your eggs, salt, and garlic powder. Grind in some black pepper.

2. Then, add in your cabbage and onion. Toss to combine.

3. In a non-stick pan, separate the mixture into 4 individual hash browns. Press them down with a spatula until they're level.

4. Cook for 3 minutes on each side until golden brown and tender.

5. I love topping mine with a fried egg and spreading the yolk generously, but you could boil some eggs instead, and chop them up while cooking the hash browns and drop that on top.

Keto Quiche With a Burrito Twist

This is the bomb, and it's spicy too. When I'm getting tired of the trusted keto quiche, I like to broaden my horizon and look beyond into the world of spices and tingling sensations. Here is the nutrition information for the keto breakfast burrito (Hunley, 2019):

Nutrition Facts	
Keto Breakfast Burrito	
Amount Per Serving (1)	
Calories 249	
	% Daily Value*
Fat 189 g	

Carbohydrates 2 g	
Fiber 0.2 g	
Protein 17.3 g	
*Percent Daily Values are based on a 2,000 calorie diet.	

What's in it:

- ½ lb ground beef

- ¼ tsp smoked paprika

- 4 oz pork breakfast sausage

- 1 tsp cumin

- ¼ cup and 2 tbsp of half-and-half

- ½ tsp chili powder

- 8 eggs

- 1 tsp garlic powder

- 1 tsp salt

- 1 cup freshly-shredded Monterey Jack cheese

Extras:

- Cilantro

- Guacamole

- Salsa

- Sour cream

Let's burrito buddy:

1. Preheat your oven to 350 °F. Grease a 9-inch cake tin with some butter or avocado oil.

2. Brown the ground beef and sausage. Break it into pieces by using your spatula, and let it brown for about 4–5 minutes until all the pink is gone.

3. Spice it up by sprinkling in your paprika, salt, garlic powder, cumin, chili powder. Mix the spices in thoroughly.

4. Whisk the eggs and half-and-half.

5. Topple the meat mixture into your cake tin, and then pour the egg and half-and-half mixture into the meat mixture mix.

6. Top with shredded cheese.

7. Bake for a good 30–35 minutes or until the cheese is a mouthwateringly brown and crispy.

8. Let it rest for 5 minutes, and chow down.

Topping

1. For a full burrito feel, you can top the slices with cilantro, salsa, sour cream, and good old guacamole.

Lunches

Many lunch favorites are already keto-approved, though you may just need to remove a few ingredients. Salads, soups, and sandwiches are easy to adjust to the *Big to Small* keto plan. Below are some classic recipes with a familiar, yet keto-friendly taste.

Lunch Box 1

This is an all-in-one kind of deal. You either go hard or go home and eat your salad. A great lunch box is a bento-style one with five separate sections, which is one of my favorite quick boxes. I find them helpful, especially if your food is in a bag and being shuffled around throughout the day.

What's in it:

- Bacon

- Hard-boiled eggs

- ½ smashed avocado

- Mozzarella sticks or string cheese

- French onion dip

Lunch Box 2
What's in it:

- Cashews

- Cheese cubes

- Blueberries

- Boiled egg with some spring onion sprinkles

- Ham roll ups

Lunch Box 3
What's in it:

- Chopped chicken filet or smoked salmon

- Cheese circles

- Cherry tomatoes

- Steamed and flavored broccoli

Lunch Box 4
What's in it:

- 3 slices of deli turkey with 3 slices of cheese rolled in them

- ½ avocado

- Cucumber slices

- Blueberries

- Almonds

Italian-Style Chicken Meatballs

These are a great, time-saving meal. You can make them for dinner the night before or pop them into your lunchbox for work. They're wonderful because you get the deliciousness of a meatball without the red meat. So, you don't have to decide between the hearty rib eye or the massive meatball. Here is the nutrition information for the italian-style meatballs (Aobadia, n.d.):

Nutrition Facts

Mozzarella cheese meatballs

Amount Per Serving (4)

Calories 150

	% Daily Value*
Fat 11 g	17%
Carbohydrates 2 g	1%
Protein 12 g	
Vitamin A	10%
Calcium	8%
Iron	10%

*Percent Daily Values are based on a 2000 calorie diet.

What's in it:

- 1 lb ground chicken or turkey
- ¾ cup shredded parmesan cheese
- 1 egg

- ½ tsp ground black pepper

- 1 tsp garlic powder

- ½ tsp dried basil

- 1 tsp salt

- 3 tbsp olive oil or avocado oil

- 1 ¾ cups boiled and peeled whole tomatoes

- 2 tbsp finely-chopped fresh parsley

- 6 ½ cups fresh spinach

- 2 oz butter

- 1 ½ cups fresh mozzarella cheese

Let's get rolling:

1. Pop the ground chicken, parmesan cheese, egg, salt, and spices into a mixing bowl, and mush it together with your hands, spreading the spices evenly.

2. Roll your meaty mixture into balls of about 1 ounce each. Keeping your hands wet helps roll them out nicely.

3. Heat up your oil of choice in a large skillet, and sauté your meatballs until brown all over.

4. Turn the heat down a bit, and add your chopped and peeled boiled tomatoes. Let it sit for 15 minutes, simmering away. Stir every few minutes.

5. Season it with some salt and a little pepper, and then add the parsley. Stir afterwards.

6. In a separate pan, melt your butter, and fry the spinach for 1–2 minutes.

7. Add the spinach to the meatball mix. Stir to combine.

8. Sprinkle mozzarella over the top, and dig in.

Lunch Box 5
What's in it:

- 3 cooked chicken meatballs

- Zoodles—zucchini noodles—tossed with olive oil and lemon juice

- Cubed cheddar cheese

- Roasted almonds

- Babybel cheese circles

Cobb Salad

Salads have long been a light, fresh meal to keep you powered through the day. However, the cobb salad contains so many keto-friendly ingredients, your taste buds will be unable to keep up. This convenient meal is packed into one bowl and drizzled with delicious, healthy dressing. Choose a dressing with minimal ingredients and that is, preferably, oil-based to keep it healthy.

What's in it:

- 1 boiled egg

- 2 strips pan-seared bacon

- ¼ cup diced tomato

- 1 cup lettuce

- ¼ cup diced cucumber

- A sprinkle of shredded cheese

- ⅛ cup diced red onion

- 2 tbsp dressing

What to do:

1. Simply toss it all together and enjoy!

BLT Lettuce Wrap

Wraps are a popular lunch option, and by removing the tortilla or bread for lettuce, you can turn almost any traditional recipe into a keto one. Additionally, lettuce leaves for a wrap can leave room for other ingredients. Create new variations of this simple food to entice your taste buds. Pair a wrap with a side of steamed and diced sweet potato or other vegetables to round out the meal.

You will need:

- 1 leaf romaine lettuce

- 2 strips thinly-sliced bacon

- ¼ tomato sliced

- 1 tbsp avocado oil mayonnaise

- 1 thin slice cheddar cheese

Directions:

1. Cook bacon in a pan until you reach the desired level of brown. Pat dry to remove excess oil.

2. Rinse the lettuce leaf, then pat it dry as well.

3. Smear avocado mayonnaise on the lettuce leaf, then place bacon, tomato, and cheese.

4. Wrap tightly, and enjoy with a side of your choice.

Gazpacho Soup

Soup at its simplest is excellent for the keto diet due to its creative use of many vegetables and spices. Gazpacho is a traditional dish from Spain and includes both fruits and vegetables in a delicious combination that's sure to inspire other soups.

You will need:

1. 4 medium-sized, vine-ripe tomatoes for liquifying

2. 3 medium-sized, vine-ripe tomatoes for peeling and dicing

3. ½ cucumber

4. ¼ cup red onion

5. 1 clove garlic

6. ½ red bell pepper

7. 2 tbsp avocado oil

8. A sprinkle of pink Himalayan salt

9. A sprinkle of black pepper

10. Blender

11. Medium-sized pot

12. ¼ jalapeno pepper—optional

What to do:

1. In a medium-sized pot, bring water to a boil. Put all tomatoes in the water for about 2 minutes, then remove them and place them in an ice bath.

2. Once the tomatoes have cooled, you will need to separate the ones for liquifying and blending. After separating them, peel and deseed them. A tip for deseeding is to put a strainer over a bowl, and squeeze the tomato. Everything that falls into the strainer will be discarded, and you will use all the juices left below.

3. Next, put the 4 tomato remnants for liquifying into the mix, and blend until it is a liquid; leave this on the side.

4. Next, dice the remaining tomatoes, and set them aside.

5. Take half the cucumber, peel it, deseed it, dice it, and set it aside. Next, dice up a ¼ cup of red onion, and set it aside.

6. Cut and deseed half a red pepper, dice it, and then set it aside with the other ingredients.

7. Now, combine all ingredients and mix in the blender with the liquid tomato. You want to leave the soup slightly thick, so don't blend for too long. Once combined into a good consistency, let the soup cool for a few hours or overnight. This recipe will yield about 2 servings.

Dinners

Dinners are known for having creative, hearty, and comforting foods, all of which you do not have to give up with a keto diet. Save your meat and carb rations for evening meals so you can recreate favorite dishes with keto ingredients.

Tomato and Avocado Skillet Shrimp

I personally adore shrimp. It's flavorful, tender, and the easiest fish group to start you on your seafood journey if you're not so keen on fish. Here is the nutrition information for the shrimp skillet (Meal Prep on Fleek, n.d.):

Nutrition Facts
Shrimp Skillet
Amount Per Serving (4)
Calories 208

	% Daily Value*
Fat 9 g	
Saturated Fat 5 g	
Carbohydrates 6.5 g	
Fiber 1.7 g	
Sugars 3.6 g	
Protein 24.5 g	
Vitamin A 1,012 IU	
Calcium 179 mg	
Iron 2.72 mg	
*Percent Daily Values are based on a 2,000 calorie diet.	

What's in it:

- 2 tbsp ghee
- 1 lb peeled shrimp
- Salt and pepper
- 4 chopped scallions
- 1 avocado
- ½ tsp dried parsley

- 3 cloves minced garlic

- 1 tbsp lime juice

- 1 lb diced and seeded tomatoes

- 1–2 tsp chipotle peppers

- ¼ cup freshly-chopped cilantro

What to do:

1. Heat your ghee up on a skillet over medium to high heat.

2. Season the shrimp with the parsley, salt, and pepper.

3. Flip them into the skillet with a sizzle. Cook them for 1 minute to keep them tender.

4. Add your tomatoes, scallion, garlic, and chipotle.

5. Cook everything until the shrimps are opaque.

6. Take them off the stove, and pop in the avocado, lime juice, and cilantro.

7. Place on a plate, and enjoy.

Keto Lasagna

Lasagna has been one of my favorite dishes since I was a child as my mom makes the best lasagna. I try to keep it as a staple meal for my family as well. With an astounding net carb total of 4 grams, this is a no-brainer for treat day. Here is the nutrition information for the keto lasagna (Tasha, 2016):

Nutrition Facts	
Lasagna Keto Style	
Amount Per Serving (4)	
Calories 544	
	% Daily Value*
Fat 41 g	63%
Carbohydrates 6 g	2%
Fiber 2 g	8%
Sugars 3 g	3%
Protein 34 g	68%
*Percent Daily Values are based on a 2,000 calorie diet.	

What's in it:

- 16 oz chicken mince, or beef if you can

- 1 cup Rao's marinara sauce

- 10 oz ricotta cheese

- 4 oz shredded mozzarella cheese

- 1 large zucchini

What to do:

1. Preheat the oven to 350 °F.

2. Peel your zucchini into thick strips, then put some salt on them. Let them sit for 15 minutes.

3. While waiting for the zucchini, you can brown the meat in a saucepan. Once the meat is brown, you can pour in the marinara sauce and season with salt and pepper.

4. Place a layer of meat and sauce.

5. Then, place a layer of zucchini.

6. Atop the zucchini, place a nice thick layer of ricotta.

7. Do a couple of layers of the zucchini and ricotta.

8. Top with mozzarella.

9. Cover with foil, and bake for 30 minutes.

10. Then, remove the foil and grill for 2–3 minutes to brown the cheese.

Fried Chicken

Crunchy, savory, and delicious are all things you want and will get from this recipe. The process is not all that different from traditional, non-keto recipes. The main differences are that you will bake rather than fry and only utilize keto-friendly ingredients and spices.

You will need:

- 1 chicken breast, skinless

- Pink Himalayan salt

- Pepper

- 1 egg

- ¼ cup heavy cream

- ½ cup almond flour

- ½ tsp garlic powder

- ¼ tsp paprika

- Baking pan

- Aluminum foil

Directions:

1. Rinse off the chicken in cold water, and set it aside.

2. Preheat the oven to 400 °F.

3. Grab a couple of small bowls. In one, combine spices and almond flour, then mix well.

4. In the other bowl, crack open the egg, add the heavy cream, and whisk together with a fork to create an egg wash.

5. Now, dip the chicken in the egg wash, and pat it around in the flour mixture. Make sure all of the chicken is covered.

6. Next, place the chicken on an oven-safe pan. Put the chicken in aluminum foil to save yourself cleanup work after you're done. Keep the chicken baking for

about 45 minutes or until the outside is golden brown.

Zucchini Taco Boat Recipe

Using vegetables as a substitute for bread is a great way to enjoy your favorites while on the keto diet. This recipe pulls on the classic taco night but replaces the tortilla with zucchini to keep the traditional spice flavors at the forefront.

What's in it:

- 1 zucchini

- ½ cup ground beef, 5–10% fat only

- ½ bell pepper

- ¼ cup shredded cheese

- 2 tbsp salsa—be wary of too much sugar and preservatives

For seasoning:

- ½ tsp cumin

- ½ tsp chili powder

- ½ tsp oregano

- ¼ tsp garlic powder

- ¼ tsp onion powder

- ¼ tsp paprika

- A dash of pink Himalayan salt

- A dash of pepper

- Baking pan

- Aluminum foil

Directions:

1. Preheat the oven to bake at 400 °F.

2. In a pan, brown the beef.

3. Once brown, add the bell peppers, seasoning, and a bit of water to help mix the ingredients.

4. On the side, cut the stem off the zucchini, and then cut it in half lengthwise. Carve out the inside, and store it for future recipes. Sprinkle a bit of salt on the zucchini, then fill each half with the beef mixture.

5. Next, sprinkle the shredded cheese on top of the zucchini, and place it in the oven on an oven-safe pan with aluminum foil. Once the zucchini has softened and the cheese has melted, pull it out of the oven.

6. Top each half with a tablespoon of salsa, and enjoy. Feel free to add sliced avocado on top if daily intake requirements allow.

One Pan Lemon Chicken

There's nothing better than a meal with limited dishwashing afterwards. This is also a great summertime mix up, and you have an opportunity to get that leon in there. This dish is simple, delicious, and even great the next day with some avocado mayonnaise. You could even pop the mixture onto flaxseed crackers. Here is the nutrition information for the lemon chicken (Nevins, 2017):

Nutrition Facts	
Lemon Chicken	
Amount Per Serving (4)	
Calories 298	
	% Daily Value*
Carbohydrates 7 g	
Fiber 2 g	
Sugars 2 g	
Protein 35 g	
*Percent Daily Values are based on a 2,000 calorie diet.	

What's in it:

- 2 tbsp olive oil

- 4 chicken breasts, with skin

- 1 lb asparagus

- 2 cloves garlic

- 1 cup chicken stock

- 1 tbsp fresh chopped parsley

- ½ zest of lemon

- 3 tbsp lemon juice

What to do:

1. Pound your chicken pieces by placing them between two pieces of plastic wrap and giving them a good whack with a tenderizer or rolling pin.

2. In a large pan, add your olive oil, and bring it to a medium-high heat. When it's nice and toasty, drop in the chicken breasts, and cook each side for about 5 minutes or until golden brown.

3. Take them out the pan and put them to the side. Then, toss your asparagus into the pan, and sauté for 1 minute.

4. Drop in your garlic, and sauté for another minute.

5. In a bowl, whisk together the lemon juice and mustard until fully mixed. Pour the mixture into the asparagus with the stock as well. Sprinkle in the zest too.

6. Bring the liquid to a boil, and then let simmer for 3–4 minutes while covered.

7. Uncover it, and let that scented steam rise. Stir in the parsley, and add the chicken back into the pan.

8. Rotate the breast to cover it in sauce, and then it's ready to go.

Lemon and Rosemary Salmon

Herbs and meat are meant to be together on a plate. While this recipe may not be new, it is an example that utilizing classic seasonings and meats can keep the keto diet fun.

You will need:

- 1 salmon piece
- ½ lemon, sliced
- 1 tbsp rosemary
- 1 tbsp coconut oil
- ½ tsp pink Himalayan salt
- ½ tsp pepper
- Oven-safe pan
- Aluminum foil

Directions:

1. Preheat the oven to bake at 400 °F.

2. Wrap the oven-safe pan in aluminum foil, and set it aside.

3. Arrange half of the lemon slices on the pan where you will be placing the salmon.

4. In a small bowl, mix the oil and herbs.

5. Coat the salmon evenly with the mixture, place it on the pan, and top with the remaining lemon slices.

6. Put it in the oven for approximately 20 minutes or until the fish is thoroughly cooked.

Not So Sneaky Snacks

Snacks are shunned in diet culture for adding unnecessary calories to your daily limits. Fortunately, keto works to keep you satisfied and your body in fat-burning mode, so you'll need to incorporate some snacks. The *Big to Small* keto plan suggests two small snacks throughout the day and an optional evening snack. Something as small as six cashews and a handful of blueberries can be considered a snack, but for those who want a little more for this small meal, there are a couple of recipes below. Here is the nutrition information for the keto mint bars (Ketchum, 2021):

No Bake Keto Mint Bars

Nutrition Facts	
No Bake Keto Mint Bars	
Amount Per Serving (1 Bar)	
Calories 259	Calories From Fat 221
	% Daily Value*
Fat 24.6 g	38%

Carbohydrates 6.3 g	2%
Fiber 3.1g	12%
Protein 3.5 g	7%
*Percent Daily Values are based on a 2,000 calorie diet.	

You're going to need:

Crust

- ⅓ chopped pecans

- ⅔ cup shredded coconut

- 1 cup almond flour

- 1 tsp vanilla extract

- 1 large, slightly beaten egg

- 6 tbsp Swerve Sweetener—powdered

- ⅓ cup cocoa

- ½ cup butter

Filling

- 4 oz softened cream cheese

- 1 cup powdered Swerve Sweetener

- ½ cup softened butter

- 2 tsp peppermint extract

- Natural green food coloring

- 2 tbsp heavy whipping cream room temperature

Chocolate Glaze

- 3 oz chopped sugar-free dark chocolate

- 2 tbsp butter

Let's build from the bottom up—crust:

1. You're going to place a medium saucepan onto your stovetop which will be on a low heat to allow the butter to melt slowly. Sieve in the cocoa powder and sweetener, and then gently whisk in the egg so it doesn't cook too quickly or unevenly.

2. Stir the mixture until the mixture thickens. Take it off the stovetop, and then mix in your vanilla, almond flour, shredded coconuts, and those delicious nutty pecans.

3. Grab a 9x9 or 8x8 square pan and pour your mixture into it, pressing down the filling until it's even. Then, pop it into the fridge until it's firm. It should take about 20 minutes. So, get to making that filling.

Let's do the green bit—filling:

1. Grab a large bowl that can catch your spray of cream cheese and butter. Then, beat your cream cheese and butter, and add in the sweetener. Keep beating it until it's all blended. Remember to beat it gently without overbeating it.

2. Drizzle the peppermint extract over the creamy, buttery mix. Then, add your whipped cream and food coloring. Mix it just enough to turn it a lovely mint green. Take into account the aesthetics while making this recipe.

3. Then, enjoy the satisfying pouring of the filling over the base. Pop it into the fridge for about 30 minutes or until firm.

Let's get to the juicy topping—chocolate glaze:

1. Place a heatproof bowl over a simmering pot of water to warm it up. Sprinkle in your chopped up chocolate, plop in some butter, and let it all smelt together. When it's a rich, creamy mixture, you can grab the almost-complete keto mint squares and layer it over the top for a snapping, texture-adding chocolate top.

If you're feeling feisty—optional garnish:

1. If you want to spruce up the squares with a fancy green drizzle, then this will be a fun addition. You should make it quick though; melt the white chocolate alongside your chocolate topping melt.

2. You might appreciate the added look when you're digging through the fridge for your post-workout treat. So, in another simmering pot, place your heatproof bowl and topple in the white chocolate pieces with some cocoa butter. Stir it until it's smooth and rich.

3. After you have topped your filling with the chocolate glaze, trickle on the white chocolate mixture in straight lines.

4. With a toothpick, create perpendicular lines by dragging the toothpick across the white lines. It should look like a cross forming tiny chevrons in the white lines.

Now, you can take a sneaky piece and cut up the rest to keep in the fridge for your next moment of weakness, but do try to keep the munchies to a minimum.

Flaxseed Crackers

They're amazing for taste and because of the nutritious and healthy flaxseeds. It's also a great snack if you're really craving carbs. Here is the nutrition information for the crackers (VanNewhyzen, n.d.-b):

Nutrition Facts	
Crackers	
Amount Per Serving (4)	
Calories 258	
	% Daily Value*
Fat 20 g	
Carbohydrates 1.25 g	

<table>
<tr><td>Protein 9 g</td><td></td></tr>
</table>

*Percent Daily Values are based on a 2,000 calorie diet.

What's in it:

- 1 cup ground flaxseed

- 5 tbsp chia seeds

- ½ cup water

- ¼ tsp pink Himalayan salt

- 1 tbsp rosemary

- 1 tbsp black pepper

- Parchment paper

What to do:

1. Preheat your trusty oven to 375 °F.

2. Line a large baking tray with parchment paper.

3. In a mixing bowl, pour in the chia seeds, flaxseeds, and spices. Mix it well so the flavor is evenly spread.

4. Slowly pour in ½ cup of water. Keep mixing it as you add the water, and stop when it's a firm, doughy consistency.

5. Scoop it up, then drop it onto the parchment paper. Layer it out by using a nice flat spatula or spoon.

6. It's important to get them as even as possible because they're crackers. It will also mean no burnt edges or soggy bits.

7. Make thin lines in the dough about cracker size to make it easier to break up when it's done.

8. Bake for 30 minutes, but check it frequently to avoid burning it.

9. Remove it from the oven, and let it cool completely.

10. Break them into crackers, and enjoy with a keto-friendly dip.

Minty Chocolate Smoothie

There is nothing more to say. This is just pure bliss. Here is the nutrition information for the mint chocolate smoothie (Tripkovic, 2020a):

Nutrition Facts	
Mint Chocolate Chip Smoothie	
Amount Per Serving (1)	
Calories 241	
	% Daily Value*
Fat 13.7 g	21%
Saturated fat 1.7 g	9%

Carbohydrates 10.7 g	4%
Fiber 6.3 g	25%
Sugars 1 g	
Protein 18.5 g	

*Percent Daily Values are based on a 2,000 calorie diet.

What's in it:

- 1 ½ cup unsweetened almond milk
- 2 cups spinach
- ½ chopped avocado
- 1 scoop chocolate keto protein powder
- ¼ cup fresh mint leaves
- 1 tbsp chopped dark chocolate

What to do:

1. Plug in that blender, and pop the lid.

2. Toss in the spinach, avocado, protein powder, and mint leaves.

3. Blend on high speed until it's juicy and thick. You could also add some ice cubes if you'd like it a little cooler.

4. Pour into a glass, and drop some dark chocolate chips on top.

5. Guzzle down immediately.

Spicy Avocado half
What's in it:

- ½ avocado

- A sprinkle of pink Himalayan salt

- A sprinkle of pepper

- 2 tsp hot sauce

- ½ tbsp avocado oil mayonnaise

Directions:

1. Cut the avocado in half, and save one half for use later.

2. Use a fork or knife to cut into the avocado. Make it into slices.

3. Next, sprinkle the salt and pepper lightly.

4. Mix the avocado oil, mayonnaise, and hot sauce in a bowl or leave them separate.

Baked Cinnamon Banana Slices

After a good workout, enjoy this snack to satisfy your sweet cravings. Plain fruit will always be a good choice for a snack, but it's fun to give it a twist every once in a while. Be inspired to adjust it to your preferences, and create unique fruit recipes by leaving the fruit cold or frozen and using other keto-friendly spices.

You will need:

- ½ banana, sliced about a ¼-inch thick

- 1 tbsp coconut oil

- 1 tsp cinnamon

- Baking pan

- Aluminum foil

Directions:

1. Preheat the oven to bake at 400 °F, and put aluminum foil on the pan.

2. Peel and cut a banana in half. Save one half for later by freezing it; this will help it last longer.

3. Mix the coconut oil and cinnamon in a bowl. Using a spoon or brush, smother the banana in the mixture.

4. Bake for about 10 minutes, adjusting the time based on how soft you want the banana to get. Let it cool, slice it, sprinkle a little more cinnamon on top, and enjoy.

Must Make Brownies

I don't think I need to say more. Who doesn't love brownies? Here is the nutrition information for keto brownies (Abraham, 2020):

Nutrition Facts
Keto Brownie

Amount Per Serving (1)	
Calories 260	
	% Daily Value*
Fat 23 g	
Saturated fat 9 g	
Carbohydrates 11 g	
Fiber 5 g	
Sugars 1 g	
Protein 7 g	
*Percent Daily Values are based on a 2,000 calorie diet.	

What's in it:

- 2 tsp vanilla extract
- ½ tsp kosher salt
- ⅔ cup cocoa powder
- ⅔ cup Swerve Sweetener—keto-friendly, granulated
- 2 tsp baking soda
- 6 tbsp peanut butter
- ½ cup peanut butter

- ½ cup melted butter

- 2 ripe avocados

- 4 large eggs

What to do:

1. Preheat that oven to 350 °F.

2. Line an 8x8 inch square pan with parchment paper.

3. In a blender or food processor, combine all of the ingredients. Blend until thick and smooth.

4. Pour the batter into the baking pan, and smooth it with a flat spatula. The rubber ones really are the best.

5. Bake for 25–30 minutes or until the brownies are soft but not wet. You can use a toothpick to check the inside. It should come out dry.

6. Let them cool for 25–30 minutes, and enjoy your delicious keto brownies.

Beverages

It is hard to think of what you are drinking as adding to your weight, but what you drink each day plays an important role in your weight loss. First and foremost, there are no sugary drinks, which cuts many lifelong favorites out. The key to the perfect, keto-friendly beverage is finding no-calorie flavors to combine with water. Although that may sound limiting, there are hundreds of drinks you can have that way, such as flavored seltzer water, teas, coffee, and fruit-infused waters. Below, you will find a few recipes of some drinks you can make at home with simple ingredients.

Green Tea

Green tea is a delicious drink you can have any time of the day. This beverage has no calories, but it has multiple benefits. Green tea boosts energy levels, speeds up your metabolism, lowers your heart rate, and helps your body burn fat away.

You will need:

- 8 oz water

- 1 bag green tea leaves

- Mug

Directions:

Heat the water in the mug in the microwave for 2 minutes or until the water is steaming. Place the green tea bag into the mug, and let it steep for about 2 minutes. Let the tea cool to your desired temperature and enjoy.

Lemon Water

While not necessarily a recipe, lemon water made it to the list because of its uses. When your body is dealing with withdrawals from sugars and processed foods, you may get a headache. Drinking some lemon water will help subside the pain.

You will need:

- 8 oz water

- ½ fresh lemon

- Cup

Directions:

Fill the cup with water at any temperature. Squeeze the lemon juices into the water or let it steep.

Sample Daily Menu

This will be an example of a daily menu based on someone who exercises for a minimum of 30 minutes, 4 times per week. This menu is only a suggestion to demonstrate how meals, drinks, and snacks are broken up throughout the day.

Breakfast:

- Oat bowl

- Green tea

- 16 oz water

- 100 mg vitamin C supplement

Midmorning snack:

- Pear

- 6 almonds or any other nut you may like

Lunch:

- ½ chicken breast or turkey steak

- Vegetable stir fry—fried in coconut oil—on a bed of raw spinach

- Green tea

- 16 oz water

Dinner:

- Omelet—2 large eggs stuffed with a vegetable cooked in coconut oil

- Turkey bacon cooked in coconut oil

- Green tea

- 16 oz water

Bedtime Snack:

- 2 tbsp full-fat Greek yogurt

- ¼ cup blueberries

- 1 tbsp chia seeds

Please note that it's suggested that you consume 32 ounces of water for every 50 pounds you weigh.

Chapter 4: Let's Get Physical—Exercise Routines

Putting in the hard work in the kitchen is only part of the battle ahead. Physical exercise will ensure you burn more calories than you're consuming, guaranteeing weight loss. Hundreds of routines and machines exist for exercise, but at the end of the day, you will need to find what works for you and motivates you.

Try a combination of every exercise listed below to help pass the time and work every inch of your body. For example, cardio will help burn fat fast, so utilize it to drop the most pounds within three weeks. Likewise, weight-intensive workouts will help burn fat and replace it with muscle to help you begin carving out that perfect physique.

Regardless of what exercises you choose, make sure to be safe. Your body is going to be experiencing a lot of changes mentally, physically, and even emotionally. Do not underestimate the need for a slower-paced routine as you adjust. This plan will help you drop weight, not transform you into the next gold medal Olympian. Sticking to the dietary restrictions and exercise routines are bragging rights enough in our book.

My number one rule is to limber up or lose your workout. There are countless benefits to stretching before and after workouts. It mostly helps with recovery and preventing injuries because of tight muscles. Stretching also allows for a mindful moment before your workout, so you can connect with your body and your muscles. It increases your range of motion, keeps your muscles limber, improves posture and joints, and becomes more important as you age. If you've ever experienced a sprained ankle or torn quadricep, then you'll understand the importance of stretching. Plus, the more you do it, the more flexible you will be, and life in general will just be easier and more comfortable. Keep in mind that you can also stretch incorrectly, so pay attention to your body and your breathing while you're stretching.

Best Stretches

This is a 10-minute, quick stretch you should do before and after any workout. But, as you become more flexible and strong, then you can up your game and get to a yoga class!

Lying Hamstring Stretch

Lay down on your back, preferably on a mat or towel. Lay with both legs straight out and your body in line. Then, simply lift one leg perpendicular to your body and hold onto the back of your thigh while you breathe into the stretch and enjoy the release. Keep your core engaged, and hold the stretch for a good 20 seconds. Do the same with the other leg.

Ankle To Knee

Staying on your back brings both your knees up by sliding your feet closer to your bum. Lift your right foot and place your right ankle on your left knee. Keep your back against the ground, and breathe into the pose for at least 20 seconds. Swap legs, and repeat.

Lying Torso Twist

Lay flat on the ground again with your body relaxed, and take a deep breath. Then, bring your left knee towards your chest and over your body to your right side. Stretch your left arm out to the opposite side of your leg, and enjoy that stretch. Hold for 20 seconds and then swap sides. You should basically be twisted but don't continue if you feel any sharp pains.

Downward Dog

Get onto your hands and knees with your shoulders directly above your hands. Keep your spine neutral in tabletop position. Tuck your toes and lift your knees, bringing your tailbone up to the sky. Be sure to get that V-shape and keep your back straight with your core tight. Hold for 20 seconds, and don't forget to breathe into those stretching muscles.

Plank

For this one, you'll get onto your hands and toes as straight as possible. Use that core to keep you up and keep your shoulders engaged.

Cobra

Lay flat on your front. Then, place your hands next to your shoulders with your forearm alongside your body. Simply push through your elbows and forearms and lift the top half of your body off the ground.

Runners Lunge

Get onto your feet, and step forward with one foot. Lower yourself until your hands are on either side of your front foot. Descend until your knee is as close to the ground as possible. Tilt your pelvis forward, and squeeze those glutes. Hold for 20 seconds. Then, swap sides.

Shoulder Stretch

Stand up nice and straight, and simply stretch your right arm across your body to the left side, holding your right elbow with your left hand. Breathe into the stretch, and hold for 20 seconds before switching sides.

Tricep Stretch

Stand up straight or sit down, but your back must be straight. Then, put your right hand on your right shoulder, and use your left hand to slowly push your right elbow up. Hold for 20 seconds, and move onto the other arm.

Heart Racing Cardio—No Machines, Just You

Cardio exercises will get your heart rate up and your fat levels down as you sweat the pounds away. It focuses on increasing your heart rate, typically through routines without weights, and is the best exercise choice for those on a tight schedule or budget. It gets your body moving enough to help shed weight in many different ways, with or without gadgets.

Cardio is the most straightforward exercise because it doesn't require any sort of machinery, memberships, or particular locations. All you need is an able body and motivated mindset. Simply walking will increase your heart rate and have you complete cardio exercise to fuel weight loss. For many, simple exercises are not enticing, so it's necessary to move in a way that makes you enjoy the activity. Below are a few exercises that do not require equipment other than yourself and appropriate workout clothing. Some ideas to make the activities engaging and the typical calories burned will be included.

Walking

Consider walking in a plain, black T-shirt as it's simple and goes with everything. Take a walk around a parking lot, a track, the mall, the neighborhood; the list goes on and on where you can utilize this activity. Find a beautiful park with incredible scenery or an inside area with air conditioning to add pleasure to this simple task. Walking requires less concentration than other exercises and maintains a slower pace so you can let your mind wander as you go. Before you know it, 30 minutes will have come and gone.

A 30-minute walk at a pace of a mile every 17 minutes for a 155-pound person burns approximately 133 calories.

Running

What running is all about is an exercise that will get the heart pumping and the sweat pouring. Running has many benefits, from improving your endurance to acting as a means of stretching your legs. It may require more space to roam, but a 30-minute run on a beautiful spring day is as good as it gets. Inspire yourself to run by joining a marathon training group or aiming to set a new personal record within the 3-week timeframe.

A 30-minute run at a pace of a mile every 12 minutes for a 155-pound person burns approximately 288 calories.

Swimming

Who needs to sweat and overheat when you could splash around in a pool? Swimming submerses you into another element and allows you to move your body in a unique way. While no one expects you to set the next Olympic pace, try pushing yourself to set a new lap record. Add extra variety to this exercise by opting for a combination of indoor or outdoor pools. Also, morning and evening swimming always feel different, so it's hard to find a reason not to keep swimming fun.

A 30-minute swim in general for a 155-pound person will burn approximately 216 calories.

Dancing

A little shake here and shimmy there, dancing is easily one of the most versatile exercises. Join a local class, or stay home, put on a favorite playlist, and let loose. As long as you move your body to the beat, or not, since this is a judgment-free space, the calories are burning. Motivate yourself by trying to learn a new dance style or perfect the one you already know.

A 30-minute, low-impact dance session for a 155-pound person will burn approximately 198 calories.

Pedals to the Metals: Machine-Based Cardio

Equipment-based cardio is convenient whether you go to a public gym space or have the machines at home. Play your favorite television shows, movies, podcasts, or playlists as 30 minutes breeze by. Additionally, machines are engineered to target specific muscles and muscle groups safely. Listed below are cardio machines that target different parts of the body.

Row Machine

Feel the benefits of a fast-paced boat trip from the comfort of a sliding seat. The rowing machine will work your shoulder and arm muscles so you can build a little definition while keeping up that heart rate. Up the resistance of the chain, or rope, to push your body. Keep this exercise exciting by imagining a fun Viking adventure or setting a new record.

A 30-minute session on the rowing machine for a 155-pound person will burn approximately 252 calories.

Treadmill

A legend in the exercise equipment world, the treadmill allows for some of the simplest yet dynamic workouts. Hold some dumbbells as you briskly pace in place. Maybe emulate one of those classic Hollywood movie scenes and watch the morning news with a slight incline and moderate speed. Treadmills will work the same muscles as walking, primarily leg muscles and some back ones. So, there are few reasons to get bored of a treadmill and its numerous possibilities.

A 30-minute walk on the treadmill is the same as a walk; a 155-pound person will burn approximately 133 calories.

Stairclimber

Ascend to the skies—or at least 10 feet closer—as you walk endless steps toward a thinner you. The stair climber will work your calves, thighs, and glutes while having you sweat like you've been running. Use this machine to work specific muscles by changing the part of your foot you step with or by changing how many stairs are in between each step. Keep the exercise interesting by setting new paces and records over the weeks.

A 30-minute, average-paced workout on the stair climber for a person who weighs 155 pounds will burn approximately 216 calories.

Bicycle

Live out your Tour de France dreams or childhood memories with a sedentary bicycle. Going nowhere, this bike will surely take you a few pedals closer to weight loss as your heart gets pumping. Challenge yourself to set a faster pace, and feel the calf and thigh muscles get a great workout. If your arms are tired, this is the perfect way to give your upper body a break.

A 30-minute stationary bike workout for a 155-pound person will burn approximately 252 calories.

Heavier Weights, Lighter You

No one can be upset about getting a more toned, muscular frame. We're not talking about being a heavyweight champion but putting some definition into your figure. Lifting weights accelerates your heartbeats per minute and targets particular muscles and muscle groups for growth.

If you're not interested in building muscle, don't worry about feeling like you missed something. Muscle growth does not necessarily equal increased weight loss. The amount of calories it takes to keep the body running when muscles are present is higher than leaner builds. Simply put, muscles require more calories to maintain daily function but are not necessary for dropping weight.

For those interested in exercising a bit more strenuously, below are some easy, weighted exercises to use in combination. We suggest doing 20 repetitions of each exercise in 3 sets, but you can adjust them as needed. Although it's not impossible, doing a single weighted exercise for 30 minutes straight isn't helpful. Instead, try incorporating as many as possible into a 30-minute session without losing your energy and strength. For someone who weighs 155 pounds, 30 minutes of adequate weight lifting will burn approximately 108 calories.

Upper Body

Bench press

Working out and laying down—who knew they went together? This classic exercise which focuses on your chest, biceps, triceps, and deltoids will make your upper body look great. Start at a feasible weight that challenges you. By the end of the third repetition, you should feel some muscle pain that lasts for a minute or two.

Bicep curl

Watch out. Your arms will become guns after working these muscles! Bicep curls will turn an ordinary workout into a 1980's montage moment. Try alternating curls to challenge yourself, and work out in front of a mirror to boost your ego as you watch those biceps flex.

The Lawnmower

Get ready for spring grass cutting by engaging your shoulder, tricep, and side muscles in this fun exercise. Grab a bench or find a flat surface. Put your leg on the floor, and rest the opposite knee on the bench with the hand on the same side as your propped-up leg. Next, grab a dumbbell with your free hand, which should be on the same side as your foot on the floor, and lift the weight up to your side. Keep your elbow close to your side, and bring your hand even to your chest. Repeat this exercise 20 times, repeat 3 times, and increase the weight by 5 or 10 pound increments.

Seated Pull Down

A classic back workout is a seated pull-down which comes in a variety of machines. The one similarity in any of the different types of machines is a handle bar that starts in an up position that will stretch your arms out. Adjust the weight accordingly, straighten your back, lean back at a slight angle while keeping your feet planted on the floor, and pull the bar toward your chest.

Lower Body

Deadlift

Grab a bar weight or a couple of dumbbells, and rest your arms in front of you or by your side. Position your feet under your shoulders and keep the knees straight, but not so much that you push them backward. Keeping your back straight, bend forward and let the weight pull you down until you feel the tension in the back of your thighs. Now, raise your body back up to start position and repeat. Deadlifts should be done in sets of 20 and 3 cycles.

Calf raises

Multistory buildings will be no match for you after you complete this exercise. Grab a couple of dumbbells, or kettlebells, that are lighter but still heavy enough to pull your arms down. Place your feet under your shoulders. Then, lift your heels off the ground, putting all your weight on the front of your feet. When raised by your feet, your body should be straight, just as when your feet were flat on the ground. Repeat this up and down motion 20 times for 3 repetitions.

Weighted Squat

Effective, classic, and simple squats are an easy way to build muscle, and adding weights will take this exercise to the next level. A squat is only as good as the stances, so keep your feet under your shoulders. Keep your back straightened to keep the focus on your legs and not your lower back.

There are a couple of ways to go about a weighted squat, depending on your level of comfort in the gym. First, grab a kettlebell or dumbbell and hold it to your chest. The second involves more balance expertise as you rest a bench bar with weights on your shoulders. Either way, bring your butt down until your legs are as close to a 90° angle as possible. Then, repeat that motion 20 times and for 3 repetitions.

Leg Press

Feel like a superhero in this fun machine to work all your legs, glutes, thighs, and calves. First, adjust the seat, catch bar, and weight level to your approval, and push the platform up and down. For better results, bring your knees as close to your chest. Additionally, the further apart you position your legs, the more your inner thighs will be worked. Next, adjust the height of your footing to work more on the front or back of your legs. Last, for a bonus calf workout, position just the front of your foot on the platform, and push up and down.

Chapter 5: Cheat Day and Challenges

Everyone deserves to treat themselves after 2 weeks of pushing boundaries and changing their routine. For keto, that means you will get to eat and drink however and whatever you want for a joyous 24 hours. While not a limitation, it is suggested you try to keep your eating schedule and portion sizes the same as the diet. Enjoy all the foods you have been dreaming about because they're finally yours to devour.

Cheat Day, Oh Yay!

While eating the foods you were unable to, notice how your body reacts to the ingredients you have deprived yourself of. Your digestive system and routine bodily functions have been running on lighter ingredients with the careful intention behind them. In cleansing your system of preservatives, sugars, carbs, and other "heavy" ingredients, your body will have acclimated to healthier foods, and reintroducing them for one day will be an excellent opportunity to assess your regular diet. Think about what foods may make you feel tired, sick, or otherwise not well. Though the diet is meant to help you lose weight, learning about your body during the diet is more important for long-term health.

Not So Fast

Did you think we would let you get away with all that cheating? The day after your cheat day, I ask that you practice intermittent fasting for 24 hours. You are still permitted to drink water, green tea, or lemon water anytime during this day, but you should only consume approximately half your usual calories; supplements are also welcomed.

Eating that slowly through the day or in one meal is up to you. Your body should have more than enough nutrients to last you through the day, but you know your body best. If for any reason you have to eat, keep it to a minimum and follow the keto-approved items.

Willpower

Food is more than an energy source for our bodies; it brings about emotions and unconscious behaviors. Putting yourself on the keto diet will test your physical limit with hunger and working out as well as your mental ability to continue with the *Big to Small* keto plan when your body is asking for more. These bodily demands may look like cravings, exhaustion, body pains, and many other subliminal messages. Sticking to the diet in the face of these discomforts requires more internal strength than external.

First, knowing your typical shortcomings with mental battles will be essential. For example, hunger may not bother you, but a headache could push you over the limit. Additionally, think about your relationship with food. Do you reward yourself after an accomplished goal, or, on the other hand, do you grab a sweet treat after a hard day? Maybe the shortcoming has nothing to do with your behavior but everything to do with pressure from family and friends to go out to dinners or drinks where there are little to no healthy keto options. Awareness is key when dealing with personal battles, meaning you must know your enemy to defeat them.

Second, you will need to develop habits, tricks, or anything else to avoid or face your mental battles. Sure, preventing or stopping the behavior is the most straightforward answer, but you must be realistic with yourself. You are much more likely to break the diet by adding additional stress; save that fight for another day. In the case of rewarding yourself with food, maybe reward yourself with inedible treats instead. Treat yourself to a 30-minute break for shows or videos, or buy a new item that you've been putting off. The possibilities are endless.

In the same way that friends or family can sway your success, they can also help you achieve it. Whether you're beginning or already familiar with the keto diet, find a confidant with whom you can share your daily concerns and achievements. Allowing someone else to know what you're feeling and thinking will allow for intervention when necessary and praise when earned.

Time

The keto diet, when properly followed, will require a lot of time and effort from its participants. Researching recipes, cooking, and working out are only surface-level examples of time-consuming chores that need to be done each day. When faced with a typical yet busy life, adding additional steps can feel overwhelming. To make the timing work, you may sacrifice sleep, other responsibilities, and eventually, even the diet. Although you cannot turn back the clock, there are a few simple hacks to help buy you some time.

Meal prep

Most people will find that a day or two during their week allots them more free time than other days. On those days, utilizing that precious time to prepare meals for the week will save much more time throughout the week. Decide on a favorite recipe or ingredient, and cook it in bulk. Those foods can then be stored in the refrigerator and freezer to use later in the week. If you find that preparing entire meals in advance leads to wasted food, try preparing ingredients you are sure to utilize. You can cut up certain fruits, vegetables, meats, and grains with little seasoning, allowing you to decide on the flavor later. After the first few days, you'll quickly see which ingredients you do or don't use, helping you build a better shopping list and schedule.

Find simple recipes

Ambition can be your downfall in the kitchen. Sure, a made-from-scratch cauliflower pizza dough sounds delicious and would allow you to indulge in a food you miss, but is it possible with your timetable? Luckily, the keto diet is aimed toward small quantities of ingredients, but there are lots of recipes that will take even less time. Remember that seasonings and your choice of oil will add so much extra flavor to a dish that you may not need to use many ingredients to begin with. Words like "quick," "simple," or "few ingredients" may be necessary for your recipe searches.

Multi-task

Help free up some of your time now taken over by keto by multitasking. For example, that new episode of the latest bingeable show can be done while you prepare and cook your meals. Listen to that book you wanted to read while cutting up the ingredients. Multitasking with the proper technique can allow the keto diet to merge with your daily and weekly routines seamlessly.

Budget

Getting the best necessary ingredients, spices, and supplements can be a real challenge for your wallet. Looking at restaurant menus and the organic section of produce, it is reasonably evident that eating clean is not the cheapest decision. It doesn't make much sense to stick to a diet that you cannot afford to begin with. Understanding how to bargain shop and substitute flavors will be vital to saving money.

Bargain budget

There are many different avenues to finding cheaper options. First, there are numerous brands of any item in most stores, which gives the shopper the advantage. Pay close attention to the ingredients list on the differently priced foods. If the two products have a similar ingredient list, then it's acceptable to go with the cheaper option. A final tip will add a step to your grocery planning trip, but it will be worth it: Go to the websites of the various grocers in your area and look for sales. While on the websites, you can typically check prices as well. Locating the best deal and comparing store prices will help you stay within your budget.

Flavorful finances

Elaborate sauces and recipes can construct some of the best dishes in the world while demolishing your wallet. Knowing how to make less food just as satisfying and recreating flavors of ingredients will save you a little cash. Opt for powdered spice or liquid versions of a food's taste when needed. Also, knowing the substitutes or ingredients of favorite sauces or tastes can help.

For example, let's say that you enjoy dishes with soy sauce in them. Through a bit of research, you can discover that soy sauce is preferred for offering a salty, sweet, and bitter taste. Look in your cabinets; you may find you already have salt, sugar, and some vinegar. While these ingredients may not directly replace the taste of soy sauce, you can experiment with doses of each until you build a similar taste or at least cater it to your liking. Lastly, selecting more straightforward recipes with flavorful meats and produce can help lower the shopping bill.

Additional Recommendations

For those who aren't seeing the results they wanted or those who want to push themselves a little harder, here are some recommendations for various parts of the plan.

When planning your day, try to put your heaviest meal around the middle of the day. By eating the fatter foods in the middle of the day, you allow your body to use up more of that energy before bedtime. Since the workouts are only 30 minutes, it will be easy to find a time in the morning or late afternoon to still incorporate your carbs in the meal closest to your workout.

Try going vegan during the keto diet to help you lose more weight. By not using meat and dairy products, you will lower your calorie and carb intake. Protein comes in various plants or nuts and the necessary nutrients can be taken with supplement pills or powders. Dairy provides fats and other vitamins that you can acquire from items already recommended in the *Big to Small* keto plan.

Conclusion

Deciding to lose weight is a big decision because it will require a change in your lifestyle, not just your meals. The *Big to Small* keto plan incorporates exercise and eating while also refraining from alcohol. These steps will require commitment, practical recipes, shopping, and drive. Although it will require effort, it doesn't have to be arduous work. The plan is flexible in many parts and is designed to be as easy or as difficult as you would prefer. Additionally, since the plan is designed to only last for three weeks, it's also something that can be repeated as many times as you want. Losing weight and achieving your health goals will feel effortless, all thanks to the *Big to Small* keto diet plan.

References

Abraham, L. (2019, February 7). *Best-ever cabbage hash browns.* Delish. https://www.delish.com/cooking/recipe-ideas/a26044120/cabbage-hash-browns-recipe/%20https://www.delish.com/cooking/a1192/how-to-cook-tofu/

Abraham, L. (2020, December 23). *Keto brownies.* Delish. https://www.delish.com/cooking/nutrition/a58586/keto-brownies-recipe/

Allen, B. G., Bhatia, S. K., Anderson, C. M., Eichenberger-Gilmore, J. M., Sibenaller, Z. A., Mapuskar, K. A., Schoenfeld, J. D., Buatti, J. M., Spitz, D. R., & Fath, M. A. (2014). Ketogenic diets as an adjuvant cancer therapy: History and potential mechanism. *Redox Biology, 2,* 963–970. https://doi.org/10.1016/j.redox.2014.08.002

Aobadia, A. (n.d.). *Italian keto meatballs with mozzarella cheese.* Diet Doctor. https://www.dietdoctor.com/recipes/keto-italian-meatballs

Basmati rice vs. Brown rice. (n.d.). Old School Labs www.oldschoollabs.com/basmati-rice-vs-brown-rice/#:~:text=Based%20on%20the%20nutrition%20information

Berg, E. (2017, April 3). *Why lemon juice is essential on a ketogenic diet.* Dr. Berg. https://www.drberg.com/blog/why-lemons-are-essential-on-a-ketogenic-diet#the

Berg, E. (2019, October 15). *Dr. Berg's healthy keto basics: Start here.* Dr. Berg. https://www.drberg.com/blog/healthy-keto-plan-start-here

Boost your cholesterol-lowering potential with phytosterols. (n.d.). Cleveland Clinic. https://my.clevelandclinic.org/health/articles/17368-phytosterols-sterols--stanols

Brazier, Y. (2017, November 27). *What you need to know about acne.* Medical News Today. https://www.medicalnewstoday.com/articles/107146#causes

Bryant, R. (n.d.). *Avocado benefits: The keto dieter's best friend.* Ketogenicinfo. https://ketogenicinfo.com/avocado-keto-benefits/#:~:text=One%20of%20the%20benefits%20of%20avocado%20on%20keto

Chef Sky Hanka. (2021, October 7). *Fully loaded keto breakfast parfait recipe.* Trifecta. https://www.trifectanutrition.com/blog/fully-loaded-keto-breakfast-parfait-recipe

Cohut, M. (2020, January 23). *'2–3 oz of walnuts' daily may benefit heart and gut health.* Medical News Today. https://www.medicalnewstoday.com/articles/waln

uts-may-be-good-for-the-gut-and-help-promote-heart-health#Just-how-healthful-are-walnuts

Bueno, N. B., de Melo, I. S. V., de Oliveira S. L., & de Rocha Ataide, T. (2013, May 7). Very-low-carbohydrate ketogenic diet v. low-fat diet for long-term weight loss: a meta-analysis of randomised controlled trials. *The British Journal of Nutrition. 110*(7), 1178–1187. https://doi.org/10.1017/S0007114513000548

Calories burned in 30 minutes for people of three different weights. (2021, March 8). Harvard Health Publishing. www.health.harvard.edu/diet-and-weight-loss/calories-burned-in-30-minutes-for-people-of-three-different-weights

Can you eat dandelions? (2021, July 2021). Cleveland Clinic. health.clevelandclinic.org/dandelion-health-benefits/

Chia seeds. (n.d.). Harvard T.H. Chan. www.hsph.harvard.edu/nutritionsource/food-features/chia-seeds/

Dandelion. (n.d.). Mount Sinai. www.mountsinai.org/health-library/herb/dandelion#:~:text=Fresh%20or%20dried%20dandelion%20herb

8Fit Team. (n.d.). *Full-body stretching routine: 10-minute guided session.* 8fit. https://8fit.com/fitness/full-body-stretching-routine-10-minute-guided-session/

Eske, J. (2019, December 5). *Melatonin: Is it safe for babies?* Medical News Today. https://www.medicalnewstoday.com/articles/3272 24#about-melatonin

Harguth, A. (2022, 21 March). *What you should know about processed foods.* Mayo Clinic Health System. www.mayoclinichealthsystem.org/hometown-health/speaking-of-health/processed-foods-what-you-should-know

The health benefits of eggs. (n.d.). Australian Eggs. www.australianeggs.org.au/nutrition/health-benefits

Health benefits of hemp seeds. (2018, September 11). Medical News Today. www.medicalnewstoday.com/articles/323037

Is MCT oil worth the hype? (2021, December 28). Cleveland Clinic. health.clevelandclinic.org/mct-oil-benefits/

Gore, M. (2020, December 18). *Keto cereal.* Delish. https://www.delish.com/cooking/recipe-ideas/a25238263/keto-cereal-recipe/

Gore, M. (2021, December 21). *Gluten-free pop tarts.* Delish. https://www.delish.com/cooking/recipe-ideas/a32715418/gluten-free-pop-tarts-recipe/

Gunnars, K., & Streit, L. (2022, April 12). *7 enticing health benefits of Chia seeds.* Healthline. https://www.healthline.com/nutrition/11-proven-health-benefits-of-chia-seeds#TOC_TITLE_HDR_3

Hamzic, H. (2020, April 24). *10 keto smoothie recipes that are so refreshing.* Kiss My Keto. https://blog.kissmyketo.com/articles/food/keto-smoothie-recipes/#:~:text=Ketogenic%20smoothies%20can%20be%20made%20with%20things%20like

Healer Admin. (n.d.). *The endocannabinoid system.* Healer. https://healer.com/blog/the-endocannabinoid-system/

Hunley, A. (2019, May 9). *Keto breakfast burrito quiche: Meal prep and freezer meal.* Keto in Pearls. https://ketoinpearls.com/keto-breakfast-burrito-quiche-meal-prep-and-freezer-meal/

Ketchum, C. (2021, September 16). *Keto mint chocolate bars.* All Day I Dream about Food. https://alldayidreamaboutfood.com/keto-mint-chocolate-bars/#recipe

Ketogenic diet explained. (n.d.). Charlie Foundation. https://charliefoundation.org/learn-about-ketosis/

Krampf, M. (2018, January 8). *Keto low carb green smoothie bowl recipe with spinach.* Wholesome Yum. https://www.wholesomeyum.com/recipes/keto-low-carb-green-smoothie-bowl-recipe/

Kubala, J. (2018, June 28). *The 9 best keto supplements.* Healthline.

https://www.healthline.com/nutrition/best-keto-supplements#TOC_TITLE_HDR_8

Laura. (2022, March 11). *The best keto blueberry muffins.* Delightfully Low Carb. https://delightfullylowcarb.com/keto-blueberry-muffins/

Lavado-García, J., Roncero-Martin, R., Moran, J. M., Pedrera-Canal, M., Aliaga, I., Leal-Hernandez, O., et al. (2018, January 5). Long-chain omega-3 polyunsaturated fatty acid dietary intake is positively associated with bone mineral density in normal and osteopenic Spanish women. *PLOS ONE 13*(1): e0190539. https://doi.org/10.1371/journal.pone.0190539

Link, R. & Tan, V. (2022, January 31). *The top 9 health benefits of flaxseed.* Healthline. www.healthline.com/nutrition/benefits-of-flaxseeds#TOC_TITLE_HDR_11

Mansoor, N., Vinknes, K. J., Veierød, M. B., & Retterstøl, K. (2016, February 14). Effects of low-carbohydrate diets v. low-fat diets on body weight and cardiovascular risk factors: a meta-analysis of randomised controlled trials. *The British journal of nutrition, 115*(3), 466–479. https://doi.org/10.1017/S0007114515004699

Maroon, J., & Bost, J. (2018, April 26). Review of the neurological benefits of phytocannabinoids. *Surgical Neurology International, 9*(1), 91. https://doi.org/10.4103/sni.sni_45_18

Mayo Clinic Staff. (2020a, November 13). *Whey protein*. Mayo Clinic. www.mayoclinic.org/drugs-supplements-whey-protein/art-20363344

Mayo Clinic Staff. (2020b, November 17). *Vitamin C*. Mayo Clinic. www.mayoclinic.org/drugs-supplements-vitamin-c/art-20363932

Mayo Clinic Staff. (2020c, December 8). *Fish oil*. Mayo Clinic. www.mayoclinic.org/drugs-supplements-fish-oil/art-20364810

Mayo Clinic Staff. (2021, February 9). *Vitamin D*. Mayo Clinic. www.mayoclinic.org/drugs-supplements-vitamin-d/art-20363792

McAuliffe, L. (2021, December 31). *Keto fish: The top 6 fatty fish to eat on a ketogenic diet*. Doctor Kiltz. https://www.doctorkiltz.com/keto-fish/

McCracken, M. (2018, July 10). *You shouldn't be eating meat at every meal on keto—here's why*. Brit + Co. https://www.brit.co/how-much-meat-on-keto/

McKay, D., Eliasziw, M., Chen, C., & Blumberg, J. (2018, March 11). A pecan-Rich diet improves cardiometabolic risk factors in overweight and obese adults: A randomized controlled trial. *Nutrients, 10*(3), 339. https://doi.org/10.3390/nu10030339

McKillop, J. (n.d.). *I swapped my usual snack for hemp seeds—here's how to eat them in 15 ways*. Well and Good. www.wellandgood.com/15-ways-to-eat-hemp-seeds/

Meal Prep on Fleek. (n.d.). *Skillet shrimp with tomato and avocado.* Meal Prep on Fleek. https://mealpreponfleek.com/skillet-shrimp-with-tomato-and-avocado/

Neijat, M., Suh, M., Neufeld, J., & House, J. D. (2015, October 29). Hempseed products fed to hens effectively increased n-3 polyunsaturated fatty acids in total lipids, triacylglycerol and phospholipid of egg yolk. *Lipids, 51*(5), 601–614. https://doi.org/10.1007/s11745-015-4088-7

Nevins, S. (2017, March 20). *One pan lemon chicken with asparagus.* A Saucy Kitchen. https://www.asaucykitchen.com/one-pan-lemon-chicken-with-asparagus/

Paoli, A., Rubini, A., Volek, J. S., & Grimaldi, K. A. (2013, June 26). Beyond weight loss: a review of the therapeutic uses of very-low-carbohydrate (ketogenic) diets. *European Journal of Clinical Nutrition, 67*(8), 789–796. https://doi.org/10.1038/ejcn.2013.116

Pinney, J. (2017, August 27). *Mushroom & parmesan omelette.* Julia's Cuisine. https://juliascuisine.com/mushroom-parmesan-omelette/

Prakash, S. (2020, January 29). *10 easy ways to pack a keto-friendly lunch.* Kitchn. https://www.thekitchn.com/keto-lunch-ideas-2-260359

Quinoa. (n.d.). Harvard T.H. Chan. www.hsph.harvard.edu/nutritionsource/food-features/quinoa/

Sass, C. (2021, October 27). *Are avocados healthy? 6 health benefits of the superfood.* Health. www.health.com/nutrition/avocado-health-benefits

Schiffer, S. (2016, April 21). *My favorite noatmeal (AKA lowcarb oatfree porridge): The basic recipe and 6 variations.* Healthy Sweet Eats. https://www.healthysweeteats.com/my-favorite-noatmeal-aka-low-carb-oat-free-porridge-the-basic-recipe-and-6-variations/#recipe

Seeds, hemp seed, hulled. (2019, April 1). U.S. Department of Agriculture. https://fdc.nal.usda.gov/fdc-app.html#/food-details/170148/nutrients

Sharma, R. (n.d.). *Starting strong is good. Finishing strong is epic.* QuoteNova. https://www.quotenova.net/authors/robin-sharma/x33a4v

Shoemaker, S. (2019, May 17). *The 13 best nuts and seeds for keto.* Healthline. https://www.healthline.com/nutrition/best-nuts-for-keto#TOC_TITLE_HDR_5

Suni, E. (2022, August 10). *Stages of sleep.* Sleep Foundation. https://www.sleepfoundation.org/stages-of-sleep

Tasha. (2016, October 9). *Keto lasagna with zucchini noodles [recipe].* Ketogasm. https://ketogasm.com/keto-lasagna-zucchini-recipe/

Tello, C. (2021, September 9). *6 health benefits of chlorogenic acid + side effects.* SelfDecode. https://supplements.selfdecode.com/blog/chlorogenic-acid/#:~:text=%20Chlorogenic%20acid%20may%20also%20work%20by%3A%20.

10 reasons why you should eat breakfast every day. (n.d.). Florida Milk Blog. https://www.floridamilk.com/in-the-news/blog/nutrition/10-reasons-why-you-should-eat-breakfast-every-day.stml

Tey, S. L., Brown, R. C., Chisholm, A. W., Delahunty, C. M., Gray, A. R., & Williams, S. M. (2010, September 29). Effects of different forms of hazelnuts on blood lipids and α-tocopherol concentrations in mildly hypercholesterolemic individuals. *European Journal of Clinical Nutrition, 65*(1), 117–124. https://doi.org/10.1038/ejcn.2010.200

Tindall, A. M., Petersen, K. S., Skulas-Ray, A. C., Richter, C. K., Proctor, D. N., & Kris-Etherton, P. M. (2019a, May 1). Replacing Saturated Fat With Walnuts or Vegetable Oils Improves Central Blood Pressure and Serum Lipids in Adults at Risk for Cardiovascular Disease: A Randomized Controlled-Feeding Trial.

Journal of the American Heart Association, 8(9). https://doi.org/10.1161/jaha.118.011512

Tindall, A. M., McLimans, C. J., Petersen, K. S., Kris-Etherton, P. M., & Lamendella, R. (2019b, December 19). Walnuts and Vegetable Oils Containing Oleic Acid Differentially Affect the Gut Microbiota and Associations with Cardiovascular Risk Factors: Follow-up of a Randomized, Controlled, Feeding Trial in Adults at Risk for Cardiovascular Disease. *The Journal of Nutrition, 150*(4), 806–817, https://doi.org/10.1093/jn/nxz289

Tripkovic, A. (2020a, April 23). *Mint chocolate chip green smoothie.* Kiss My Ketg. https://blog.kissmyketo.com/recipes/keto-breakfast/mint-chocolate-chip-green-smoothie/#incredients-top

Tripkovic, A. (2020b, April 23). *Strawberries & almond chocolate smoothie.* Kiss My Keto. https://blog.kissmyketo.com/recipes/keto-breakfast/strawberries-almond-chocolate-smoothie/

VanNewhyzen, P. (n.d.-a). *Are flaxseeds keto friendly? Yes, here's why!* TeamKeto. https://teamketo.com/blogs/articles/are-flaxseeds-keto-friendly/

VanNewhyzen, P. (n.d.-b). *Crunchy flaxseed crackers keto recipe.* TeamKeto. https://teamketo.com/blogs/keto-recipes/crunchy-flaxseed-crackers-recipe/

Warwick, K. W. (2020, January 8). *Is margarine more healthful than butter?* Medical News Today. https://www.medicalnewstoday.com/articles/3042 83

What is the difference between good and bad cholesterol? (2017, July 11). Keck Medicine of USC. https://www.keckmedicine.org/blog/what-is-the-difference-between-good-and-bad-cholesterol/

www.ingramcontent.com/pod-product-compliance
Lightning Source LLC
Chambersburg PA
CBHW050817260726
48660CB00004B/1487